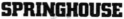
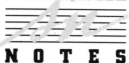

SPRINGHOUSE

N O T E S

PEDIATRIC NURSING

Janice Selekman, RN, DNSc
Dr. Selekman, the author of this book, is an Associate Professor at Thomas Jefferson University, Philadelphia. She earned her BSN from the University of Pittsburgh and her MSN and DNSc from the University of Pennsylvania, Philadelphia. Dr. Selekman is a member of the American Nurses' Association, the Pennsylvania Nurses' Association, and Sigma Theta Tau.

Jenean Hendrickson Sears, RN, MN, PhD
Dr. Sears, the reviewer of this book, is an Assistant Professor of Nursing at the University of Kansas, Kansas City. She earned her BSN and MN from the University of Kansas and received her PhD from Kansas State University. She is a member of the American Nurses' Association, Chairperson of the Research Committee of the International Childbirth Education Association, President of the Delta Chapter of Sigma Theta Tau, and a member of the American Public Health Association and the American Adult and Continuing Education Association.

Springhouse Publishing Company
Springhouse, Pennsylvania

STAFF FOR THIS VOLUME

CLINICAL STAFF

Clinical Director
Barbara McVan, RN

Clinical Editors
Lynne Atkinson, RN, BSN, CEN
Joan E. Mason, RN, EdM
Diane Schweisguth, RN, BSN, CCRN, CEN

ADVISORY BOARD

Mildred Wernet Boyd, RN, BSN, MSN
Assistant Professor, Essex Community College, Baltimore

Dorothy Brooten, PhD, FAAN
Chairperson, Health Care of Women and Childbearing Section, Director of Graduate Perinatal Nursing, University of Pennsylvania School of Nursing, Philadelphia

Lillian S. Brunner, MSN, ScD, LittD, FAAN
Nurse/Author, Brunner Associates, Inc., Berwyn, Pa.

Irma J. D'Antonio, RN, PhD
Professor and Chairperson, Department of Nursing, Mount St. Mary's College, Los Angeles

Kathleen Dracup, RN, DNSc, FAAN
Associate Professor, School of Nursing, University of California, Los Angeles, Los Angeles

Cecile A. Lengacher, RN, PhD
Director of the Division of Nursing and Health Sciences, Manatee Junior College, Bradenton, Fla.

Barbara Tower, RN, MSN, CCRN
Assistant Professor, Essex Community College, Baltimore

PUBLICATION STAFF

Executive Director, Editorial
Stanley Loeb

Executive Director, Creative Services
Jean Robinson

Design
John Hubbard (art director), Stephanie Peters (associate art director), Jacalyn Bove Facciolo, Julie Carleton Barlow

Editing
Donna L. Hilton (acquisitions), Kathy E. Goldberg, Patricia McKeown, David Prout

Copy Editing
David Moreau (manager), Edith McMahon (supervisor), Nick Anastasio, Keith de Pinho, Diane Labus, Doris Weinstock, Debra Young

Art Production
Robert Perry (manager), Anna Brindisi, Christopher Buckley, Loretta Caruso, Donald Knauss, Christina McKinley, Mark Marcin, Robert Wieder

Typography
David Kosten (manager), Diane Paluba (assistant manager), Joyce Rossi Biletz, Alicia Dempsey, Brenda Mayer, Nancy Wirs

Manufacturing
Deborah Meiris (manager),

Project Coordination
Aline S. Miller (supervisor), Maureen Carmichael

© 1988 by Springhouse Corporation, 1111 Bethlehem Pike, Springhouse, Pa. 19477. All rights reserved. Reproduction in whole or part by any means whatsoever without written permission of the publisher is prohibited by law. Authorization to photocopy items for internal or personal use, or the internal or personal use of specific clients, is granted by Springhouse Corporation for users registered with the Copyright Clearance Center (CCC) Transactional Reporting Service, provided that the base fee of $00.00 per copy plus $.75 per page is paid directly to CCC, 27 Congress St., Salem, MA 01970. For those organizations that have been granted a photocopy license by CCC, a separate system of payment has been arranged. The fee code for users of the Transactional Reporting Service is: 0874341094/88 $00.00 + $.75.

Printed in the United States of America.
SN2-011287

Library of Congress Cataloging-in-Publication Data

Selekman, Janice.
  Pediatric nursing.

  (Springhouse notes)
  Includes bibliographies and index.
  1. Pediatric nursing—Outlines, syllabi, etc.
  I. Sears, Jenean Hendrickson. II. Title.
  III. Series. [DNLM: 1. Pediatric Nursing. WY 159 S464p]
  RJ245.S37 1988   610.73'62   87-18079
  ISBN 0-87434-109-4

Contents

How to Use Springhouse Notes

Today, more than ever, nursing students face enormous time pressures. Nursing education has become more sophisticated, increasing the difficulties students have with studying efficiently and keeping pace.

The need for a comprehensive, well-designed series of study aids is great, which is why we've produced Springhouse Notes...to meet that need. Springhouse Notes provide essential course material in outline form, enabling the nursing student to study more effectively, improve understanding, achieve higher test scores, and get better grades.

Key features appear throughout each book, making the information more accessible and easier to remember.
- **Learning Objectives.** These objectives precede each section in the book to help the student evaluate knowledge before and after study.
- **Key Points.** Highlighted in color throughout the book, these points provide a way to quickly review critical information. Key points may include:
—a cardinal sign or symptom of a disorder
—the most current or popular theory about a topic
—a distinguishing characteristic of a disorder
—the most important step of a process
—a critical assessment component
—a crucial nursing intervention
—the most widely used or successful therapy or treatment.
- **Points to Remember.** This information, found at the end of each section, summarizes the section in capsule form.
- **Glossary.** Difficult, frequently used, or sometimes misunderstood terms are defined for the student at the end of each section.

Remember: Springhouse Notes are learning tools designed to *help* you. They are not intended for use as a primary information source. They should never substitute for class attendance, text reading, or classroom note taking.

This book, *Pediatric Nursing,* begins with an overview of growth and development patterns and alterations from birth through adolescence. After that, the major pediatric disorders in each section are organized by the nursing process, covering the details you'll need to remember. Such important concepts as pain in children and the effects of hospitalization are also covered. Note: Keep in mind that nursing interventions must be adapted to meet individual patient needs.

Growth and Development

Learning Objectives

After studying this section, the reader should be able to:

• Define the terms related to growth and development, and describe their impact on nursing care of children.

• Identify physical, psychosocial, and cognitive developmental tasks for children from birth through adolescence.

• Determine the nutritional and safety needs of children.

• Plan communication and other nursing interventions based on the child's needs and ability to comprehend.

I. Growth and Development

A. Concepts of growth and development

1. Growth and development are not synonymous terms
   a. Growth implies an increase in size
   b. Development describes the maturation of structures
   c. Development includes growth, but growth does not necessarily include development
2. Growth, including motor skills, and development progress as follows
   a. Cephalocaudal: head to toe
   b. Proximodistal: trunk to tips of extremities
   c. General to specific
3. Human growth is orderly and predictable; it is variable but follows a pattern
   a. Infancy: a fast growth period in which the head grows faster than other tissues
   b. Toddler/preschool stage: a slow growth period in which the trunk grows fastest
   c. School age: a slow growth period in which the limbs grow fastest
   d. Adolescence: a fast growth period in which the trunk grows again, including the gonadal and associated tissues

B. Developmental task measurements

1. Certain accomplishments are expected to be mastered during a given stage of development
2. Failure to accomplish a task may retard the development of subsequent tasks
3. Physical tasks (motor skills) include:
   a. Turning over, sitting alone, walking, writing
   b. Attainment of growth parameters
4. Erik Erikson described stages of psychosocial development (see chart, p. 17)
5. Sigmund Freud described stages of psychosexual development (see chart, p. 17)
6. Jean Piaget described stages of cognitive development (see chart, p. 17)

C. Assessments/measurements of growth and development

1. Growth charts
   a. These are recorded as percentile of height for age, weight for age, head circumference for age, weight for height
   b. Any child crossing multiple percentiles over a short period of time needs further evaluation
   c. Normal parameters are, for example:

	Birth	5 months	12 months	6 years
Height	20" (51 cm)	26" (66 cm)	30" (76 cm)	45" (114 cm)
Weight	7 lb (3.2 kg)	14 lb (6.4 kg)	21 lb (9.5 kg)	45 lb (20.4 kg)

2. Chronologic age: years or months since birth date
3. Mental age: level of cognitive function
   a. This is based on at least two intelligence tests, widely separated in time
   b. When mental age differs from chronologic age, provide toys, teach safety, and communicate based on mental age
4. Bone age: X-ray of tarsals and carpals to determine degree of ossification
5. Denver Developmental Screening Test
   a. Designed for children up to age 6
   b. Measures gross motor, fine motor, language, and personal-social development
   c. Does not measure intelligence

D. Growth and development in infancy (birth through age 1)
   1. Neonatal period (0 to 28 days of life)
      a. Head circumference equals chest circumference
      b. Head length is one fourth of total body length
      c. Brain growth depends on myelinization
      d. All behavior is under reflex control; extremities are flexed
      e. Hearing and touch are well developed
      f. Vision is poor; child fixates momentarily on light
      g. Child is stimulated by being held, being rocked, listening to music, or watching a black and white mobile
      h. Child can lift head slightly off bed when prone but not when head rests on a pillow; do not use pillows in crib
      i. Pulse normal range 110 to 160; count apically for 1 minute
      j. Respirations normal range 32 to 60; irregular; abdominal respirations; obligate nose breathers
      k. Blood pressure (BP) normal 82/46; use correct size blood pressure cuff (1.5 times diameter of extremity, or no less than half and no greater than two-thirds the length of the part of extremity being used)
      l. Temperature regulation is altered from poorly developed sweating/shivering mechanisms; decrease exposure time during bath
      m. Neonatal period has highest mortality rate
   2. Age 1 to 4 months
      a. Posterior fontanel closes
      b. Child begins to hold head up
      c. Reflexes reach their peak at 4 to 8 weeks, especially sucking, which provides nutritional, survival, and psychological pleasure
      d. At 3 months, the most primitive reflexes begin to disappear, except for protective and postural reflexes, i.e., the blink, parachute, cough, swallow, and gag reflexes, which remain for life
      e. Child observes faces and mobile, an appropriate toy for a child under age 3 months
      f. Binocular vision develops; eyes follow an object 180 degrees
      g. Child begins to put hand to mouth

    h. Reaching out is voluntary but uncoordinated; at 4 months, provide busy box on crib side or cradle gym across crib

    i. Crying expresses needs; meet needs in a consistent manner to promote trust

    j. Instinctual smile appears at 2 months; *social smile* at 3 months; social smile is child's first social response—it initiates social relationships, indicates memory traces, and indicates beginning of thought processes

    k. Child laughs in response to environment at 4 months

    l. Child regards mother's voice

    m. Child sits in infant seat (chalasia chair)

    n. Child explores his feet

3. Age 5 to 6 months

    a. Doubles birth weight

    b. Sleeps through night with one to two naps/day

    c. Begins teething (lower central incisors first)

    d. Rolls over at will

    e. When prone, can push chest up using arms

    f. When prone, uses arms to push body toward feet (creeping)

    g. Exhibits voluntary grasp and voluntary release

    h. Transfers toys from one hand to other

    i. Sits only with support

    j. Can be weaned to cup if physically and emotionally ready

    k. Cries when mother leaves; a normal sign of attachment

    l. Stranger anxiety: discerns one face from another; is wary of strangers; clings to/clutches mother

    m. Comfort habits begin: sucks thumb, rubs ear, holds blanket or stuffed toy, rocks; all habits symbolize mother and security

4. Age 7 to 9 months of age

    a. Sits alone without assistance

    b. Crawls

    c. Stands up and stays up by grasping for support

    d. Pincer grasp develops; puts everything in mouth; at high risk for aspirating objects

    e. Feeds self crackers and bottle

    f. Verbalizes all vowels and most consonants; no actual words

    g. Begins imitating expressions of others

    h. Likes his image in the mirror

    i. Develops object permanence; searches for objects outside perceptual field

    j. Discipline starts; understands the word "no"

5. Age 10 to 12 months

    a. Triples birth weight; length increases about 50% from birth

    b. Cruises (side step holding on) at 10 months; walks with support at 11 months; stands alone and takes first steps at 12 months

    c. Speaks: says mama/dada and responds to own name at 10 months; says five words but understands much more at 12 months

    d. Claps hands; waves bye-bye; enjoys rhythm games, cloth books, and toys to build with and knock over

    e. Explores everything: feels, pushes, turns, pulls, bites, smells, tests for sound

    f. Should be weaned from bottle and breast

6. Nutrition for the infant (in sequence of introduction)
   a. Formula or breast milk; no more than 30 oz (90 ml) milk/day
   b. No solid foods for first 6 months; infant doesn't physically need them and may develop allergies to foods
   c. Iron supplements after age 4 months, since iron received before birth is depleted
   d. Rice cereal is first solid food, followed by any other cereal except wheat
   e. Yellow and green vegetables
   f. Noncitrus fruits; citrus fruits after age 6 months
   g. Teething biscuits during teething
   h. Protein, i.e., eggs and meat, after age 6 months
   i. Junior foods or soft table foods after age 9 months
   j. Rules for feeding: do not put food or cereal into baby bottle (this may be recommended, though, for gastroesophageal reflux); wait 4 to 7 days before introducing a new food, to determine tolerance and potential for allergy

7. Safety tips for the infant
   a. Keep crib rails fully up at all times
   b. Use car seats properly
   c. Never leave infant unattended on dressing table; have hand on him whenever on open surfaces
   d. Always support the young infant's head
   e. Do not prop bottle while feeding
   f. Check temperature and depth (2″ at most) of bath water; keep constant hold of infant during bath
   g. Check temperature of formula and foods
   h. Remove pins, dust balls, plastic bags, etc., from infant's environment
   i. Remove hanging electrical cords; attach safety plugs to wall outlets
   j. Use gates across stairways or forbidden areas

E. Growth and development in toddlerhood (age 12 months to 3 years)

1. Introduction
   a. A period of slow growth; weight gain of 4 to 9 lb (2 to 4 kg) over 2 years
   b. Height replaces length in measuring child
   c. Normal pulse, 100; respirations, 26; BP, 99/64
   d. Vision still not mature; correction for amblyopia should be addressed at this time

2. Psychosocial development
   a. Toddlers are egocentric
   b. Child clings close to mother and now follows wherever she goes; start peek-a-boo to develop trust; progress to hide-and-seek to reinforce idea that mother will return

    c. Separation anxiety arises; bedtime is seen as desertion; fear of the dark develops

    d. Separation anxiety demonstrates closeness between child and mother; child screams and cries when she leaves, then may sulk and engage in comfort measures

    e. When mother leaves, she should announce that she is leaving but that she will return; she should leave something of hers with child; nurse should prepare mother for child's reaction and explain that this process promotes trust

    f. Transitional objects (blankets, bottles, comfort habits) represent mother and security; as long as they do not impede daily functioning and social interactions, they are not detrimental to mental health, regardless of age

    g. If child is "head-banger" or "rocker" in bed, ensure safety but ignore behavior

    h. Child may engage in solitary play; little interaction with others

3. Cognitive development

    a. Understands object permanence

    b. Engages in ritualistic behavior to master skills and decrease anxiety

    c. Has magical thinking; believes his thoughts affect events

    d. Uses symbols

    e. Finds memory enhanced by experiences; needs experiences to learn

    f. Shows curiosity about everything; not intentionally destructive

    g. Begins imitative play and role play; expresses feelings in play

    h. Lacks concept of sharing or of the value of items

    i. Can point to mentioned body parts; can recognize self in mirror

    j. Curiosity can lead to ingestion/aspiration of dangerous items

4. Mobility

    a. Focuses on exploring the environment; always active

    b. Uses arms to balance self; plants feet wide apart and walks; has flat feet; no arches. Provide push-pull toys to encourage walking

    c. Walks by age 21 months; if not, seek further evaluation

    d. At age 15 months, climbs stairs; runs and jumps by age 2; rides tricycle by age 3

    e. Has some difficulty controlling swallowing reflex and speaking

    f. Feeds self; provide finger foods

5. Dentition

    a. First molars erupt; child has 20 deciduous teeth by age 6

    b. Child introduced to toothbrush; no toothpaste yet; child just swishes and swallows

    c. Child begins using fluoride; continues until age 12

    d. Bottle mouth syndrome can be prevented by giving water in bottle or empty bottle

6. Language development

    a. Language allows child to manipulate the world with his mind; it aids perception of feelings, experiences, and memory

    b. By age 2, child uses 400 words; comprehends more than he speaks; uses two- to three-word phrases

    c. Speech is egocentric

    d. Child becomes frustrated at inability to communicate, which may result in tantrums; give more time to answer questions

    e. Age 3 is chatterbox stage; child uses 11,000 words/day

    f. Amount spoken at home influences amount a toddler speaks

    g. Child should talk by age 3; if not, seek further evaluation; assess hearing

7. Toilet training

    a. External conditions: a significant other must be committed to establishing toileting pattern, with good communication between child and adult; praise for success but no punishment for failure

    b. Internal conditions: kidneys should reach adult functioning at age 2, with mature sphincter control; child feels discomfort of wet/messy pants; child identifies elimination as cause of discomfort and recognizes sensations before excretion

    c. Toilet sitting begins at age 18 months; once every 2 waking hours; provide pleasant mood during this time.

    d. Child is physically ready when he or she removes own clothes, walks unaided, stoops/sits, talks, imitates others

    e. Child is emotionally ready when he or she acts to please others, trusts enough to give up body products, begins autonomous behavior

    f. Child may fear being sucked into toilet

    g. Child is curious about excretion products

    h. Bowel movements should not be referred to as dirty or yucky; excrement is a child's first creation; provide alternative toys, for example, clay and water

    i. With increased stress, regression may occur; toileting may have to be retaught

    j. Potty seat or potty chair should be used

    k. Underpants should be introduced to child as a badge of success and maturity

    l. Handwashing and front-to-back wiping should be taught

    m. At age 18 to 36 months, child should achieve day dryness; by age 24 to 60 months, night dryness

    n. If child isn't trained by age 5, seek further evaluation

8. Temper tantrums

    a. Child uses "no" excessively; shows assertiveness

    b. Child is curious how parent will react to "no"

    c. Child becomes frustrated; wants immediate gratification; acts out of anger; may lose control

    d. Parental intervention: provide safe environment during tantrum; identify cause; help child regain control; do not reason, threaten, promise, hit, or give in; do not tell child to wait; respond consistently; follow through on discipline free of anger

    e. Tantrum prevention: keep routines simple and consistent; set reasonable limits and give rationales; avoid head-on clashes; provide choices

    f. Overcriticism and restriction may dampen enthusiasm and increase feelings of shame and doubt

9. Safety guidelines
    a. When child starts climbing over rails of crib, switch to a bed
    b. Use locks/latches on cabinets; keep dangerous products in original containers; check plant toxicity
    c. Put pot and cup handles away from edges of table or stove
    d. Do not leave child near tubs or pools unattended
    e. Check size of toys and food particles
    f. Avoid beanbag toys (dried beans can cause instant death on aspiration)
    g. Use safety plugs in electrical outlets

F. Growth and development in preschool child (ages 3 to 5)
1. Introduction
    a. Slow growth period continues; birth length doubles by age 4
    b. Normal pulse is 90 to 100; respirations, 25; and BP, 85 to 90/60 to 70
    c. Nursery school increases contact with peers and increases incidence of infection
2. Psychosocial development
    a. Child's language is egocentric and is used to boast, brag, and shock others
    b. Child identifies with parent of same sex or primary caretaker; enjoys role-playing/modeling, dolls
    c. Child shows anxiety about health care treatments and life events (use doll play to prepare for or adjust to treatments)
    d. Child shows fear concerning body integrity (provide adhesive bandages for cuts because child fears losing all blood; anticipate fear of animal noises, new experiences, and the dark)
    e. Good sleep usually indicates good mental health
    f. Egocentricity decreases and awareness of needs of others increases; begins sharing/taking turns; attempts to please others
    g. Development of conscience and of superego begins
    h. Child becomes enculturated; learns rules; social development is enhanced by nursery school
    i. Sibling rivalry may appear
    j. Child may develop imaginary playmate to help him deal with loneliness and fears; prevalent in bright, creative children and not pathologic
    k. Disciplinary actions should be consistent; don't compare children in terms of psychosocial traits or abilities
    l. Child exhibits parallel play: activity influenced by those around him without direct interaction or sharing
3. Cognitive development
    a. Child uses three- to four-word sentences; has difficulty with pronouns
    b. Child has limited perspective but can focus on one idea at a time
    c. Awareness of racial and sexual differences begins; boys may begin to masturbate; begin sex education
    d. Child develops a body image, attaches appropriate names to body parts; parents should promote positive aspects of both sexes

     e. Concept of causality begins but child still has magical thinking
     f. Concept of time begins; parents can explain time by events; concept of today and tomorrow begins
     g. Concept of numbers, letters, and colors begins; child may count but may not understand what it means; he may recognize some letters
  4. Motor skills
     a. Dresses self, but may not tie shoes until age 5
     b. Builds towers of blocks; copies circles and lines; uses scissors; strings large beads; throws ball overhead
     c. Alternates feet on steps; hops on one foot; skips at age 5
     d. Establishes hand dominance
     e. Enjoys sandbox, water play, blocks, crayons, clay, fingerpaints
  5. Readiness for kindergarden—age 5
     a. Picks up after himself
     b. Gets along without mother for short periods
     c. Can listen and follow directions
     d. Is less afraid
     e. Speaks in correct, complete sentences

G. Growth and development in school-age child (ages 6 to 12)
  1. Introduction
     a. School shapes cognitive and social development
     b. Accidents become a major cause of injury
  2. Psychosocial development
     a. Teacher may be first major adult in child's life besides parents and may be a major influence
     b. Develops first true friendship
     c. Plays with peers: develops a sense of belonging, cooperation, and compromise; groups offer a testing ground for interpersonal interactions, the development of self-concept, and sex role behaviors; they encourage competition through fair play and relieve child of making decisions
     d. Morality develops: in early school-age, acts are right or wrong; after age 9, child understands intent and differing points of view, including gray areas; superego matures
     e. Child compares his body to others; shows modesty
     f. Child participates in family activities
     g. Awareness of societal roles begins
     h. Child engages in fantasy play and daydreaming
     i. Child may exhibit fear of death; school phobias; fear may result in psychosomatic illness
  3. Cognitive development of:
     a. Concept of time and space
     b. Concept of cause and effect
     c. Concept of nesting (building blocks, puzzle pieces)
     d. Concept of reversibility
     e. Concept of conservation (permanence of mass and volume)

      f. Concept of numbers

      g. Relationship of parts to whole (fractions)

      h. Classification of objects in more than one way

      i. Reading and spelling

      j. Interest in board games, cards; enjoys collections

4. Physical development

      a. Slow growth continues at the rate of about 2″ (5 cm) per year of height; weight doubles in 6 years

      b. First baby tooth comes out at age 6, and permanent teeth are in by age 12 except for final molars; jaw grows to accommodate permanent teeth

      c. Both sexes are same size until approximately age 9, when puberty starts for some females

      d. Bones grow faster than muscles and ligaments; therefore, children are more limber but also have more bone fractures

      e. Refinement of large and small muscle groups

      f. Vision matures by age 6

      g. Lymphoid tissue hypertrophies to maximum size

      h. Language is perfected

      i. Child participates in group activities; likes to accomplish tasks; engages in cooperative play; play involves group goals with interaction

H. Growth and development in adolescence (ages 12 to 18 +)

1. Introduction

      a. Fast growth period

      b. Vital signs approach adult values

      c. Growth consists of physical changes in body structure related to puberty, accompanied by psychosocial adjustment

2. Psychosocial/cultural development

      a. Early adolescence is spent coping with changes in physical self and becoming aware of the bodies of others

      b. Fantasy thoughts and daydreams allow role-playing of different social situations; suggest adolescent keep a diary to express feelings

      c. Middle adolescence involves exploring and identifying one's values and defining self

      d. Peers may influence fad behavior, values, or conformity

      e. Interest in opposite sex increases

      f. Late adolescence involves maturation, expressed by independence from parents, participation in society, development of self-identity, development of own morality, and planning for a future

      g. Fears at this stage include acne, obesity, homosexuality, nuclear disaster

      h. A hospitalized adolescent is in a dependent setting at a time when he should be building independence; nurse and family should provide privacy, recognize his strengths, give him as much autonomy as possible, anticipate his concerns about body image and how the illness will affect his future

3. Cognitive development
   a. Develops abstract thinking; ability to analyze, synthesize, and use logic increases
   b. Reaches adult cognitive level
4. Development of female secondary sex characteristics
   a. Hypothalamus signals pituitary to release gonadotropins; this increases secretion of leutinizing hormone (LH) and follicle-stimulating hormone (FSH), which stimulates ovarian development and production of estrogen; estrogen produces all secondary sex characteristics except axillary and pubic hair, which are controlled by adrenal androgens
   b. Breast development is first sign of puberty; begins around age 9 with bud stage; breast development takes approximately 3 years to complete and ends shortly after the first menses
   c. Fatty tissue in thighs, hips, breasts increases; hips broaden
   d. Pubic hair growth increases continuously for several years after menses begins
   e. Onset of menses occurs any time between 8th and 16th birthday; initially may be irregular
   f. Height increases up to 3″ (8 cm) per year and stops around age 16
   g. Sweat glands and sebaceous glands become more active; increased body odor and acne
5. Development of male secondary sex characteristics
   a. Hypothalamus signals pituitary gonadotropins to release LH and FSH; LH results in testicular enlargement and development of Leydig's cells in testes, which produce testosterone; FSH produces seminiferous tubules of testes, leading to spermatogenesis and fertility
   b. Testicular enlargement signals start of puberty; scrotum enlarges and penis elongates and widens; reaches adult size around age 17
   c. Muscle mass increases; chest broadens; facial and body hair proliferates; voice deepens due to growth of laryngeal cartilage
   d. Pubic hair growth increases until age 20
   e. Height increases up to 3½″ (9 cm) per year; growth stops around age 20
   f. Sweat glands and sebaceous glands become more active, increasing body odor and acne
   g. Nocturnal emissions are common; many teens who ejaculate for the first time in a nocturnal emission think they have "wet the bed"
   h. Masturbation with ejaculation is common

I. Communication with children
   1. Use words the child can understand, and explain "why"
   2. Place yourself at the child's level
   3. Never lie; tell the child when it will hurt
   4. Assess child's level of understanding
   5. Punish the child's behavior but don't threaten his self-esteem
   6. Allow the child to express his feelings fully, and respect them
   7. Communicate openly; do not ask yes-no questions unless you will accept either answer

8. When a child is hospitalized, assess his home routines and attempt to implement them where possible
9. In preparing a child for hospitalization or treatment, acquaint the child with the equipment to be used; demonstrate procedure on a doll first; teach child skills he will need after procedures; describe sensations child may experience
10. Develop a family-oriented environment; in hospital, encourage parents to participate
11. Provide play appropriate to child's mental age and disease state

J. Pain perception in children

1. Introduction
   a. Pain has physiologic and psychological components
   b. Children may associate pain with punishment
   c. Expression of pain is influenced by culture and child-rearing practices
   d. Pain thresholds vary
   e. Infants consciously withdraw from pain or pull on affected part
2. Assessment
   a. Determine intensity, type, location, duration, and circumstances of pain
   b. Assess crying, restlessness, irritability, insomnia, anger, diaphoresis, increased pulse and respiratory rate, decreased interactions, decreased appetite, fatigability, behavior changes
   c. Differentiate pathologic pain from growing pains
   d. Assess body language
3. Pain management
   a. Reinforce that pain is not punishment for misbehavior
   b. Apply comfort measures
   c. Give child a scale to grade severity of pain; give child words to describe pain
   d. Apply therapeutic touch; TLC (rub, blow, kiss, give adhesive strip bandage for minor pain)
   e. Offer distraction
   f. Administer pain medication without delay; do not minimize child's discomfort
   g. Stay with child; let child help with painful procedures to give him a sense of control
   h. After pain resolves, provide play to express feelings

THEORIES OF CHILD DEVELOPMENTALISTS

These theories should not be compared directly since they measure different aspects of development.

THEORIST	ERIK ERIKSON	JEAN PIAGET	SIGMUND FREUD
Theory Focus:	Psychosocial	Cognitive	Psychosexual
	The most commonly accepted model for child development, although it can't be empirically tested	Cognitive only; does not translate well into psychomotor skills	Serves as a precursor for more recent theories; no longer serves as the primary model
Age-groups	Ages 0 to 18 months	Ages 0 to 2	Age 0 to 6 months Oral passive (id develops; biological pleasure principle)
Infancy	Trust vs. mistrust (consistency of needs being met allows infant to predict responses to his needs)	Sensorimotor (can't learn without doing; reflexive behavior)	Age 7 to 18 months Oral aggression (teething begins; everything is put into mouth; oral satisfaction decreases anxiety)
Toddler	Ages 1½ to 3 Autonomy vs. shame and doubt (desire to do things themselves)		Ages 18 months to 3 Anal (bowel and bladder training occur; child projects feelings onto others; elimination and retention are used to control and inhibit)
Preschool	Ages 3 to 6 Initiative vs. sense of guilt (mimics; more purposeful and active in goal setting)	Ages 2 to 4 Preoperational preconceptual (egocentric, animistic, magical thinking, no cause/effect reasoning, uses symbols)	Ages 4 to 5 Phallic (ego develops [objective conscious reality], Oedipal complex—love of opposite sex parent)
School-age	Ages 6 to 13 Industry vs. inferiority (using hands to make things; being helpful; mastering tasks)	Ages 4 to 7 Intuitive/preoperational (begin cause/effect) Ages 7 to 11 Concrete operations (collections; masters facts)	Ages 6 to 12 Latent (superego develops [morality] repressed sexual drive)
Adolescent	Ages 13 to 18 Identity vs. confusion (defining self related to others)	Ages 11 to 15 Formal operations (abstract ideas; reality based)	

Points to Remember

Pediatric nursing concerns children from birth through adolescence.

All interventions are family-centered, treating the child and family as a unit.

Pediatric nursing spans the continuum from well-child care to illness and death.

Helping the child and family unit attain, maintain, and/or regain optimal health is the goal of pediatric nursing.

Health and development are affected by environment and heredity.

Motor skills develop in a cephalocaudal and proximodistal pattern.

Each stage of growth and development has specific physical, cognitive, and psychosocial developmental tasks the child should master.

Safety is an overriding concern at every stage of development.

A developmental assessment requires physical, motor, cognitive, and psychosocial parameters.

Each child is an individual with different experiences, different genes, and different reactions to life events.

Glossary

Bottle mouth syndrome—a condition caused by prolonged contact between milk/ juice sugar and enamel, resulting in decay/caries

Developmental assessment—a measurement of physical, cognitive, motor, and psychosocial parameters compared to norms for that chronologic age

Object permanence—an awareness that objects exist while not in view

Puberty—the physical changes resulting in reproductive maturity

Transitional object—an object or comfort measure that represents the security of mother

Alterations in Growth and Development

Learning Objectives

After studying this section, the reader should be able to:

- Describe the physical, psychosocial, and environmental factors that can alter growth and development.

- Plan nursing interventions to prevent deficits in growth and development and promote safety.

II. Alterations in Growth and Development

A. Failure to thrive (FTT)
1. Introduction
   a. Weight remains below third percentile; failure to gain due to either physical causes or deficient maternal-child relationship
   b. Syndrome is most frequently seen in infants
   c. If problem is related to maternal deprivation, growth and development should improve with nurturing
2. Assessment
   a. Assess for disparities between chronologic age, mental age, and bone age
   b. Assess for delayed psychosocial behavior: smiles and verbalizes little
   c. Observe for altered body posture: stiff or floppy, doesn't cuddle
   d. Review history for sleep disturbances; growth hormone is released during sleep
   e. Note rumination
   f. Review history for altered feeding techniques: bottle propping, insufficient burping
   g. Review history for altered stimulation to baby and altered knowledge of child development
3. Interventions
   a. Rule out other pathology before labeling it FTT
   b. Teach mother proper feeding and interactive techniques
   c. Help mother recognize and respond to infant's cues
   d. Act as a role model for parents
   e. Establish a structured routine and stick to it

B. Child abuse (battered child syndrome)
1. Introduction
   a. Physical or emotional abuse, neglect, or sexual abuse of child that is intentional and nonaccidental
   b. Usually indicates serious family dysfunction in communicating and coping; the child becomes the focal point
   c. May be from a poor understanding of the child's physical and psychosocial needs, resulting in unrealistic expectations
   d. Child abusers often were abused as children, and may not know healthier ways to discipline children or to show love
   e. Anyone from any social class or educational background can abuse a child; only 10% of abusers have serious psychological disturbances
   f. Abusers have low self-esteem, little confidence, and a low tolerance for frustration
   g. Toddlers are the most frequent victims
   h. Sexual abuse (referred to as "bad touch") may not be perceived as wrong at first, since most victims know and trust their abuser
2. Assessment (do not examine the child alone)
   a. Observe parent-child interactions and carefully note what the child and parents say: describe each sore, bruise, burn, and stage of healing

      b. Note if injury/symptoms fit the history of the accident/illness

      c. Note any delay in seeking help, and ask why

      d. Suspect child abuse when a child's injury doesn't match the reported accident and when X-rays show old, unexplained fractures

  3. Interventions

      a. Meet the child's immediate physical and psychological needs first, regardless of suspicions

      b. Protect the child; help the family begin to cope; try to prevent future abuse

      c. Report suspected abuse to proper authorities; this is mandated in all states

      d. Reinforce what parents do correctly; encourage their participation in child's care

      e. Teach relevant child development principles; give anticipatory guidance; serve as role model for parents

      f. Establish trust with parents and child through consistent care

      g. Engage child in play that encourages expression of feelings, especially guilt and fear

      h. Refer parents to support group

C. Accidents

  1. Introduction

      a. Accidents are the number one cause of death in children, accounting for a third of all fatalities

      b. Most accidents occur in or near the home

      c. Most accidents are preventable

      d. Safety must be a part of nursing care

  2. Common accidents in children

      a. Falls

      b. Ingestions

      c. Poisonings

      d. Drownings

      e. Motor vehicle accidents

      f. Burns

  3. Nursing interventions to promote safety

      a. Check toys for sharp edges or small pieces

      b. Anticipate motor abilities and curiosity of child

      c. Advocate use of seat belts

      d. Teach pool and bicycle safety

      e. Ensure safety in sports activities

      f. Ensure a childproof home environment: remove hanging cords, dangerous plants, all medications and cleaning agents, and block electrical outlets

      g. Supervise child's activities

      h. Teach child that pills are not candy

      i. Keep substances in original containers

4. Additional safety measures in the hospital
   a. Modify hospital environment to ensure safety based on child's mental age, developmental level, and physical condition
   b. Keep side rails on bed up at all times
   c. Avoid using friction toys when oxygen is present
   d. Avoid leaving medications or syringes at bedside
   e. Provide safety restraints, if necessary

D. Aspirin intoxication
1. Introduction
   a. Aspirin (ASA) acts as an analgesic, antipyretic, and anti-inflammatory, and inhibits platelet aggregation
   b. Normal dose is 1 grain per year of age up to age 10; peak effect occurs in 2 to 4 hours; toxicity occurs at 200 mg/kg
   c. ASA is readily available; by law, orange-flavored baby aspirin must be in small packages
2. Assessment
   a. Observe for increased respiratory rate from metabolic acidosis
   b. Note fever from stimulation of carbohydrate metabolism
   c. Note decreased blood glucose levels
   d. Assess for gastrointestinal (GI) irritation
   e. Note altered clotting function; assess for petechiae and blood loss
   f. Check for irritability, restlessness, tinnitus/altered hearing
3. Interventions
   a. Maintain patent airway; encourage hyperventilation
   b. Perform gastric lavage or induce emesis with ipecac syrup
   c. Ensure good hydration; may need calcium and potassium to flush aspirin through kidneys

E. Acetaminophen overdose
1. Introduction
   a. Acetaminophen acts as an antipyretic and analgesic
   b. Metabolized in the liver
2. Assessment
   a. Assess for GI irritability
   b. Monitor for liver damage
3. Interventions
   a. Maintain patent airway
   b. Perform gastric lavage or induce emesis with ipecac syrup
   c. Administer antidote: acetylcysteine (Mucomyst)

F. Lead intoxication
1. Introduction
   a. Obtained by teething on or eating lead-based paint or inhaling lead dust
   b. Most common in toddlers
   c. Normal blood level is 5 to 30 mcg/dl

      d. Lead is a heavy metal that is poorly absorbed by the body and slowly excreted; lead replaces calcium in bones and increases permeability of central nervous system (CNS) membranes

2. Assessment
      a. Check for bone pain
      b. Check for lead lines seen on X-rays and along gums
      c. Monitor for symptoms of anemia from inhibition of hemoglobin formation
      d. Assess for increased intracranial pressure; cortical atrophy; behavior changes; altered cognition and motor skills; seizures
      e. Check for any GI distress: constipation, vomiting, or weight loss
      f. Check for peripheral neuritis from calcium release into blood

3. Interventions
      a. Institute measures to lower blood lead level to prevent lead encephalopathy
      b. Test erythrocyte protoporphyrin to determine blood lead levels, urinalysis for coproporphyrin, and X-rays for lead lines
      c. Administer chelating agents (EDTA, BAL), which bind with lead and excrete it from body; they also remove calcium; administer deep I.M.
      d. Monitor calcium levels to prevent tetany and seizures
      e. Give large amounts of oral or I.V. fluids
      f. Discontinue iron since it binds to chelating agents
      g. Initiate referrals to discover and remove source of lead contamination

G. Burns
1. Introduction
      a. 70% of pediatric burns occur in children under age 5
      b. Burns are the third largest cause of accidental death in children, after motor vehicle accidents and drowning
      c. Under age 3, most burns result from contact with hot liquid or electricity; older children are most commonly burned by flames
      d. The rule of nines has proven inaccurate for children because head can be anywhere from 13% to 19% of body-surface area; legs are 13%

2. Assessment
      a. Assess for first-degree burn (partial thickness): dry, painful, red skin with edema; looks like sunburn
      b. Assess for second-degree burn (partial thickness): moist, weeping blisters with edema; very painful
      c. Assess for third-degree burn (full thickness): dry, pale, leathery skin; avascular without blanching or pain

3. Interventions
      a. Maintain patent airway
      b. Monitor for signs of hemorrhage
      c. Prevent and treat shock
      d. Relieve pain
      e. Care for burn wound; assist with debridement
      f. Prevent infection

H. Genetic alterations

1. General information
   a. Human cells contain 46 chromosomes in each nucleus (23 pairs); each chromosome contains thousands of genes along its deoxyribonucleic acid (DNA); chromosomes are shaped like an X
   b. Genes are the structures responsible for hereditary characteristics; they may or may not be expressed or passed to the next generation
   c. *Genotype* is the sequence and function of genes on a chromosome
   d. *Alleles* are genes of similar origin (for example, genes for eye color); homozygous alleles are identical (DD or dd); heterozygous alleles are two different alleles for the same trait (Dd)
   e. Mendel's law states that one gene for each hereditary property is received from each parent; one is dominant (expressed) and one is recessive
   f. *Karyotype* is the chromosomal pattern of a cell, including genotype, number of chromosomes, and normality or abnormality of the chromosomes
   g. *Phenotype* is the observable expression of the genes (for example, hair and eye color, body build, allergies)
   h. *Congenital* and *genetic* are not synonymous; congenital means present at birth because of abnormal development in utero (teratology); some genetic disorders may be noticeable at birth, and some may not appear for decades

2. Altered cell division
   a. Normal cell division, resulting in an exact copy of the parent cell, is called mitosis
   b. Normal cell division for procreation (reduction division), resulting in 23 chromosomes (one chromosome from each of the 23 pairs), is called meiosis (for ova and sperm only)
   c. A *mutation* is a spontaneous alteration in genes or chromosomes not present in the previous generation
   d. *Nondisjunction* is failure of one pair of chromosomes from either parent to separate during meiosis, usually resulting in 45 or 47 chromosomes in the offspring (trisomy indicates 47)
   e. *Translocation* occurs when the chromosome breaks, and parts may connect to another chromosome, or the genes may switch their order or spacing
   f. *Mosaicism* refers to different number of chromosomes in different organs of the body or a combination of the above alterations

3. Down's syndrome (trisomy 21)
   a. Usually related to nondisjunction with three chromosomes on the 21st pair (total of 47 chromosomes); risk of nondisjunction increases with increasing maternal age

    b. Assessment findings: small head with slow brain growth; upward slanting palpebral fissures (opening between eyelids); Brushfield's spots (marbling and speckling of the iris); flat nose and low-set ears; protruding tongue because of a small oral cavity; short stature with pudgy hands; simian crease (single crease across palm); hypotonia; mental age of 5 to 7 (moderate retardation)

    c. Increased risk of associated problems, for example, congenital heart defects, chronic myelogenous leukemia, and a weak immune response to infection

    d. No specific treatment for Down's syndrome beyond ordinary care for the retarded individual

4. Autosomal dominant diseases/disorders

    a. Autosomal chromosomes represent the first 22 pairs

    b. In dominant disorders, *only one* defective gene or set of genes is passed by one parent

DOMINANT DISORDERS

		affected parent	
		X	x
normal parent	X	XX	Xx
	X	XX	Xx

    c. Genetic counseling: with each pregnancy there is a 50% chance of having a child with the disease/disorder and a 50% chance of having a normal child

    d. Examples include Huntington's chorea, osteogenesis imperfecta, neurofibromatosis, night blindness

5. Autosomal recessive diseases/disorders

    a. In recessive disorders, *both* parents must pass the defective gene or set of genes to the child

RECESSIVE DISORDERS

		one parent	
		X	x
one parent	X	XX	Xx
	x	Xx	xx

    b. Genetic counseling: with each pregnancy there is a 25% chance of having a child with the disease/disorder, a 50% chance of having a child who is a carrier, and a 25% chance of having a child who is not affected

    c. Almost all carriers are free of any symptomatology of the disease

    d. Examples include cystic fibrosis, sickle-cell anemia, phenylketonuria (PKU), Tay-Sachs disease, albinism

6. Genetic sex-linked (X-linked) diseases/disorders

    a. These are associated with the 23rd pair of chromosomes

    b. Sex-linked genetic disorders are carried on the X chromosome and passed by women; women do not usually get these disorders because their other healthy X will predominate (men have no X to oppose the affected X; the Y is normally very small)

    c. Examples include baldness, hemophilia, color blindness, one type of muscular dystrophy, G-6-PD deficiency

    d. Genetic counseling: father with a sex-linked disorder has a 100% chance of passing the trait to all of his daughters, but none of his sons; however, none of his children will have the disease; in the next generation, his daughters have a 50% chance with each pregnancy of passing the disease/disorder to their sons

7. Chromosomal sex-linked disorders: Turner's syndrome

    a. Only in females: XO karotype (O represents the failure to receive one X chromosome from one parent)

    b. 45 chromosomes; no Barr body (the inactive X on the 23rd pair)

    c. Assessment findings: short stature; webbing of the neck (extra skin from ear to shoulder); low posterior hair line; low-set ears; gonadal/ovarian dysgenesis (related to nondisjunction); no sexual development or menses at puberty, low average IQ

    d. Associated cardiac and renal abnormalities

    e. Treated with estrogen to develop secondary sex characteristics and menses; sterility remains

8. Chromosomal sex-linked disorders: Klinefelter's syndrome

    a. Only in males: extra chromosome on 23rd pair, resulting in XXY (47 chromosomes)

    b. Assessment findings: failure of secondary sex characteristics to develop at puberty; tall and thin until estrogen level stimulates increased body fat distribution (especially gynecomastia); mild retardation

    c. Treated with androgens; sterility remains

Points To Remember

The nurse's role in parent education is to help promote birth, growth, and development of healthy children.

Accidents threaten the lives of children; the nurse must be a safety advocate and an educator.

The rule of nines is not applicable to pediatric burn patients because of the differences in body proportions.

Glossary

Child abuse—physical, emotional, or sexual abuse and/or neglect that is intentional and nonaccidental

Debridement—removal of eschar (dead skin) to allow granulation

Failure to thrive—weight persistently below third percentile due either to physical causes or a deficient maternal-child relationship

Rumination—voluntary regurgitation and reswallowing

Prevention of Childhood Communicable Diseases

Learning Objectives

After studying this section, the reader should be able to:

- Describe the methods of obtaining immune protection against communicable diseases.

- Describe the types of vaccines and their major side effects.

- List the schedule for suggested immunizations and its rationale.

- Describe the most common communicable diseases in children that can be prevented by immunization.

III. Prevention of Childhood Communicable Disease

A. Methods of obtaining immune protection

1. Natural/innate
   a. Present at birth; not dependent on prior contact; not learned
   b. Examples: barriers against disease, such as skin and mucous membranes; bacteriocidal substances of body fluids, such as intestinal flora and gastric acidity
   c. Some species naturally immune to some diseases
2. Naturally acquired active
   a. Immune system makes antibodies after exposure to disease
   b. Protection lasts for life
   c. High risk of side effects because child contracts disease
3. Naturally acquired passive
   a. No active immune process involved; antibodies passively received
   b. Routes: placental transfer via IgG and breast-feeding (colostrum)
4. Artificially acquired active
   a. Ingestion/injection of medically engineered substances to stimulate the immune response against specific disease
   b. Example: all immunizations
5. Artificially acquired passive
   a. Injection of antibodies without stimulation of the immune response
   b. Used as antitoxins or for prophylaxis
   c. Provide immediate protection lasting weeks to months
   d. Includes these examples: gamma globulin, a mixture of antibodies against disease prevalent in the community, pooled from 1,000 donors of human plasma; hyperimmune/convalescent gamma globulin, e.g., tetanus antitoxin, hepatitis B immune globulin, varicella zoster immune globulin

B. Types of vaccines

1. Live, attenuated
   a. Grown under poor condition, live organism results in live vaccine with reduced virulence
   b. Confers 90% to 95% protection for 20+ years with single dose
   c. Promotes full range of immunologic responses
   d. Includes these examples: measles, mumps, and rubella (MMR); Sabin polio
   e. Inactivated by heat
2. Inactivated (toxoid, killed, diffusible fraction of virus)
   a. Weaker response than live vaccines, necessitating frequent boosters
   b. Toxoid: a toxin treated with formulin or heat and rendered nontoxic but still antigenic; provides 90% to 100% protection
   c. Killed vaccine: does not promote replication; provides 40% to 70% protection
   d. Diffusible fraction of virus: part of microorganism capable of inducing immunity

C. Vaccine schedule

Immunization and route	Times of administration					
DPT (I.M.)	2 mo.	4 mo.	6 mo.		18 mo.	Ages 4 to 6
*TOPV (P.O.)	2 mo.	4 mo.	6 mo.		18 mo.	Ages 4 to 6
MMR (S.C.)				15 mo.		

Key: DPT = diphtheria, pertussis, tetanus   I.M. = intramuscularly
     TOPV = trivalent oral polio vaccine   P.O. = orally
     MMR = measles, mumps, rubella   S.C. = subcutaneously
*Every 10 years thereafter, should receive dT (one tenth the dose of diphtheria and a regular dose of tetanus)

Note: As of September 1986, the Centers for Disease Control suggests giving the DPT, TOPV, and MMR vaccines at 15 months and eliminating the 18-month booster.

1. Bacterial vaccines require at least 4 weeks between doses; viral vaccines require 6 to 8 weeks to produce peak immune response
2. Boosters for bacterial agents maintain optimal levels (titers) of antibodies by stimulating immunologic memory
   a. Primary response takes 10 to 14 days to develop an antibody titer
   b. Booster requires 1 to 3 days to reach a high antibody titer
3. Schedule for MMR vaccine is dictated by maternal antibodies; if given earlier than age 15 months, a full titer may not develop
4. All active vaccines may be administered simultaneously with different needles and at different sites
5. Active and passive vaccines are seldom given at the same time (except for tetanus), since passive vaccine can inhibit the production of a significant titer
6. If schedule is interrupted, earlier doses should not be repeated; the schedule should continue per previous guidelines
7. Immunizations should not be given earlier than the designated age
8. *Hemophilus influenzae* Type B (Hib) vaccine is recommended at age 24 months
9. Side effects and principles of vaccine administration should be noted
   a. Divided doses do not decrease the risk of side effects
   b. If child has one severe reaction, do not repeat boosters without further evaluation; ask what side effects (if any) child had from last shot
   c. Withhold pertussis vaccine if child has a progressive and active CNS problem; children with cerebral palsy can receive immunizations
   d. Do not vaccinate if child has increased temperature, since this side effect of the vaccine would be difficult to differentiate from exacerbation of original disease
   e. Do not vaccinate if child has a suppressed immune system, has received gamma globulin within the past 6 weeks, is allergic to contents of the immunization, or has been on chemotherapy
   f. Do not give tuberculosis (TB) tine test and measles immunization at the same time, since measles vaccine may make a TB-positive individual appear to be TB-negative

g. Rubella vaccine can result in arthritis 1 month after vaccination

h. Killed Salk polio vaccine (preferred for adults) can cause Guillain-Barré syndrome, seizures, or encephalopathy; oral Sabin vaccine causes polio in rare cases

D. Bacterial infections

1. Diphtheria
   a. Bacteria proliferates in respiratory tract
   b. Bacteria multiplies on dead tissue in throat, producing exotoxin and exudate consisting of a tough fibrous membrane (pseudomembrane) across respiratory tract; results in mechanical airway obstruction
   c. More serious in infants
   d. Can cause renal, cardiac, and peripheral CNS damage
2. Pertussis (whooping cough)
   a. Bacteria proliferates in respiratory tract
   b. Possibility of death from pertussis decreases with increasing age
   c. Characterized by paroxysmal/spasmodic cough that ends in a prolonged inspiratory whoop
   d. Can cause seizures, anoxia/apnea, mental retardation, hernia, stroke, pneumonia, or death
3. Tetanus (lockjaw)
   a. Anaerobic spore-forming bacteria produces an exotoxin, which is present in soil, house dust, animal feces
   b. Introduced through skin; reaches axons of nerves, causing contraction of voluntary muscles, muscular rigidity, and painful paroxysmal seizures
   c. First symptoms: trismus (lockjaw) and difficulty swallowing
   d. Can cause laryngospasm, respiratory distress, intramuscular hemorrhage, or death
   e. No transplacental immunity; attacks are equally dangerous in adulthood and in childhood
   f. If clean wound is less than 6 hours old with immunizations less than 5 years old, no treatment is needed; if clean wound and immunizations less than 10 years old, give toxoid; if dirty wound and initial series is not complete or if immunizations are more than 10 years old, give toxoid and immunoglobulin
4. *Hemophilus influenzae* Type B (Hib)
   a. Leading cause of serious bacterial disease in U.S. (bacterial meningitis, epiglottitis, sepsis, cellulitis)
   b. 25% are older than 24 months; this is only group helped by vaccine
   c. Rarely spread on environmental surfaces
   d. Give vaccine after age 24 months; no boosters since no immune memory is induced (T-cell independent)

E. Viral infections

1. Rubeola (measles)
   a. Respiratory tract virus lasting 10 days
   b. Begins with prodromal symptoms: fever, malaise, harsh rasping cough, conjunctivitis, coryza

    c. Disease symptoms: maculopapular, red, pruritic rash; photophobia; Koplik's spots on buccal mucosa

    d. Can cause bacterial superinfections, such as encephalitis with possible retardation; death; subacute sclerosing panencephalitis

2. Rubella (German measles)

    a. Respiratory tract virus lasting 3 days

    b. Symptoms: subauricular and suboccipital lymphadenopathy; pink, mild maculopapular rash

    c. Rubella can cause arthralgia/arthritis, idiopathic thrombocytopenic purpura, encephalitis

    d. Congenital rubella syndrome is seen in infants whose mothers contracted rubella during pregnancy; results in growth and mental retardation, cataracts, deafness, cardiac anomalies

3. Parotitis (mumps)

    a. Respiratory tract virus

    b. Symptoms: swelling in parotid glands and painful swallowing

    c. Can cause aseptic meningitis, orchitis, and epididymitis in older males; nerve deafness; encephalitis

4. Poliomyelitis (polio)

    a. Fecal-oral virus that replicates in the GI tract and then enters blood

    b. Symptoms: initially, stiff neck and muscle pains; nerve cell damage; asymmetrical flaccid paralysis; no sensory deficits

    c. Three types of polio can occur; all in trivalent oral polio vaccine (TOPV)

    d. 30 to 40 years after illness, patient may develop postpolio syndrome with muscle weakness

5. Varicella (chicken pox)

    a. Respiratory herpes zoster virus; no protection from maternal antibodies

    b. Highly contagious from 2 days before rash to 6 days after rash; incubation period is 21 days

    c. Symptoms: vesicular pruritic rash beginning on trunk; vesicles crust and scab

    d. Scabs are not infectious; child may return to school when all lesions have scabbed

    e. Interventions include keeping nails short; patting, not rubbing, sores; applying calamine lotion; giving cool starch or oatmeal baths; administering antihistamines; dressing child in light, loose-fitting clothes

    f. Can cause bacterial superinfections, pneumonia, ataxia, encephalitis, Reye's syndrome, shingles

F. Rickettsial infections: Rocky Mountain spotted fever

1. Tick-carried rickettsia
2. Symptoms: rash with cardiovascular and CNS involvement
3. Remove tick by grasping with tweezers close to point of attachment and pulling slowly and steadily; by using tissues to pull tick out; or by covering tick with petroleum jelly

Points to Remember

Naturally acquired active immunity lasts longest but has the highest risk of side effects because child contracts disease; artificially acquired active immunity via immunizations is preferred.

The immunization schedule depends on whether antigen is viral or bacterial, on the level of titer produced, on the length of time the titer is maintained, and on factors that interfere with titer development.

Acquainting consumers with the complications of communicable diseases and with the potential side effects of vaccines will instill trust and ease society's fear of immunizations, thus increasing the number of children protected.

Glossary

Attenuated—live vaccines grown under suboptimal conditions to reduce virulence

Immunization/vaccination—injection/ingestion of antigen that promotes formation of antibodies against a specific disease

Incubation period—period between reception of antigen and initiation of clinical symptoms

Toxoid—a toxin rendered nontoxic

Altered Hematologic Functioning

Learning Objectives

After studying this section, the reader should be able to:

• Describe and differentiate among conditions involving alterations in red blood cell, white blood cell, and platelet function.

• Assess and plan care for children who are anemic and immune-suppressed and who have clotting deficiencies.

IV. Altered Hematologic Functioning

A. Basic concepts
1. General information
   a. All five blood cell types are made in bone marrow and originate from the same stem cell (see page 36)
   b. Early in utero, all blood cells are made by the liver and spleen; these organs retain some hematopoietic ability throughout life
   c. Before birth, the bone marrow becomes the main producer of blood cells
2. Blood composition
   a. Cellular portion includes erythrocytes (red blood cells), thrombocytes (platelets), and three types of leukocytes (white blood cells): lymphocytes, monocytes, and granulocytes
   b. Plasma portion is largely water; it also includes plasma proteins, electrolytes and dissolved nutrients, clotting factors, anticoagulants, and antibodies
3. Functions of blood
   a. Respiration
   b. Nutrition of body cells
   c. Excretion via transport of wastes to other organs
   d. Maintenance of acid-base balance
   e. Regulation of body temperature
   f. Defense against foreign antigens
   g. Transport of hormones

B. Altered red blood cell (RBC) functioning
1. Introduction
   a. RBCs transport oxygen from lungs to tissues and carbon dioxide from tissues to lungs
   b. Reticulocytes are precursors of mature RBCs; they comprise 2% of total RBCs and predict RBC production
   c. RBCs live 120 days; at death, most of their iron is conserved; the remaining products produce indirect bilirubin; liver enzyme converts indirect bilirubin to direct bilirubin so it can be excreted in bile
   d. RBC production is stimulated by erythropoietin in response to hypoxia
   e. Erythropoietin is made in the kidney
   f. Excess RBC production is called polycythemia
   g. Newborns normally have a high RBC count
   h. Hemoglobin (Hb) is the iron-containing pigment in RBC; it carries oxygen to body tissues
   i. RBCs are described by size (macrocytic, microcytic, normocytic) and color (hyperchromic, hypochromic, normochromic)
2. Normal hemoglobin changes
   a. During first 6 months of fetal life, 90% of hemoglobin is HbF (fetal hemoglobin), which absorbs oxygen at a lower tension; at birth, 75% of Hb is HbF

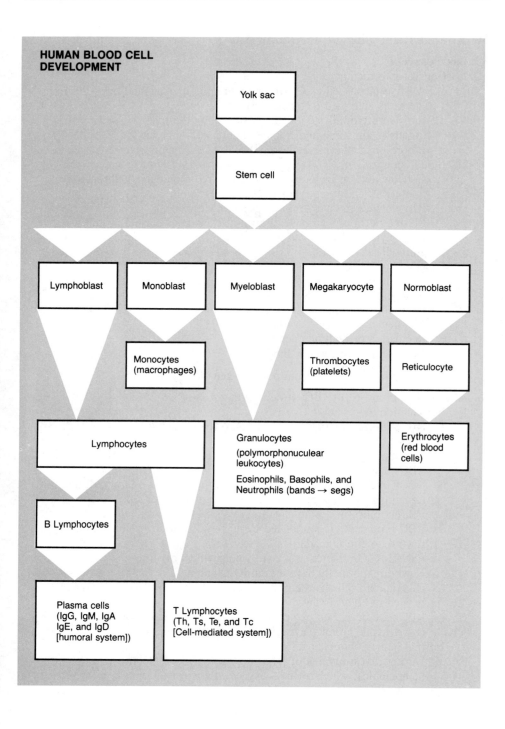

HUMAN BLOOD CELL DEVELOPMENT

Yolk sac

Stem cell

Lymphoblast

Monoblast

Myeloblast

Megakaryocyte

Normoblast

Monocytes (macrophages)

Thrombocytes (platelets)

Reticulocyte

Lymphocytes

Granulocytes (polymorphonuculear leukocytes)

Eosinophils, Basophils, and Neutrophils (bands → segs)

Erythrocytes (red blood cells)

B Lymphocytes

Plasma cells (IgG, IgM, IgA IgE, and IgD [humoral system])

T Lymphocytes (Th, Ts, Te, and Tc [Cell-mediated system])

b. Production of adult hemoglobin (HbA) begins during last 2 months in utero; it slowly replaces HbF and reaches adult levels by age 2

c. Infants' Hb level is lowest between age 4 and 6 months, when HbF is decreasing and HbA is developing; this state is called *normal physiologic anemia*

C. Anemia

1. Introduction
   a. A red blood cell disorder
   b. The most common hematopoietic disorder of childhood
   c. A symptom rather than a diagnosis
   d. Anemia may be from decreased production or life span of RBCs, decreased size of RBCs, or decreased amount of hemoglobin
   e. Anemia may also be from acute or chronic blood loss, increased RBC destruction, decreased production of RBCs from bone marrow depression, or the absence of substances needed to make RBCs

2. Assessment
   a. Take diet history; document nutrients needed to make RBCs
   b. Note patient malnutrition or anorexia
   c. Check for drug use (phenytoin [Dilantin], nitrofurantoin [Furadantin], sulfa) that would interfere with RBC production
   d. Check urine, stool, and emesis for blood
   e. Note pallor from tissue hypoxia
   f. Note skin breakdown from poor oxygenation of tissues
   g. Check for jaundice and pruritus from large amounts of unconjugated bilirubin in the blood related to hemolysis of RBCs
   h. Note increased pulse and respirations as body compensates for hypoxia
   i. Note altered neurologic status/behavioral changes from poor oxygenation of the brain
   j. Assess for hepatomegaly and splenomegaly from sequestered RBCs related to hematopoietic and phagocytic functions of liver and spleen
   k. Note weakness or low exercise tolerance
   l. Note growth retardation
   m. Review history for frequent infections, common in anemia
   n. Note gum hypertrophy and smooth tongue

3. Interventions for all anemias
   a. Determine and eliminate cause
   b. Decrease oxygen demands: plan activities; provide passive stimulation; allow frequent rest; give small, frequent feedings with soft foods; elevate head of bed
   c. Implement good handwashing and mouth care
   d. Maintain normal body temperature

4. Additional interventions for iron deficiency anemias
   a. Provide foods high in iron (liver, dark leafy vegetables, whole grains)
   b. Administer iron before meals with citrus juice because iron is best absorbed in an acidic environment; give oral liquid iron with a straw to prevent staining of skin and teeth

D. Aplastic anemia
1. Introduction
   a. Failure of bone marrow to produce RBCs and other blood components
   b. A congenital or acquired condition, frequently due to an autoimmune process
2. Assessment
   a. Prepare for and assist with bone marrow aspiration in iliac crest; diagnosis confirmed by abnormal results
   b. Assess for symptoms of anemia plus symptoms of platelet deficiency (see "Altered clotting function," page 40) and white blood cell deficiency (see Section V, "Altered immunologic functioning")
3. Interventions
   a. Administer cortisone regimen to stop autoimmune process
   b. Prepare for possible bone marrow transplant

E. Spherocytosis
1. Introduction
   a. A hemolytic anemia
   b. Abnormal rigidity in membrane structure of RBCs
   c. RBCs are spherical instead of biconcave; cannot change shape as needed
   d. Spleen traps cells and destroys them, causing hemolytic anemia
2. Assessment
   a. Note symptoms of anemia
   b. Assess for splenomegaly
   c. Note jaundice from large amounts of unconjugated bilirubin in the blood related to large numbers of destroyed RBCs
3. Intervention: spleen removal

F. Beta-thalassemia/thalassemia major/Cooley's anemia
1. Introduction
   a. A hemolytic anemia
   b. Production of beta chain of HbA is impaired, resulting in normal RBCs with decreased amounts of Hb
   c. Production of HbF increases to compensate for decreased HbA
   d. RBCs are more fragile; fail to hold oxygen well, are easily destroyed, and have a very shortened life span
   e. Hemolysis increases, releasing hemosiderin, which deposits in the skin; skin appears bronze (hemosiderosis)
   f. Increased hemolysis also releases unused iron, which can build up in heart muscles, causing heart failure
   g. As bone marrow attempts to compensate for anemia, hyperplasia of bone marrow cavity and thinning of bone marrow cortex may occur; bone pain, pathologic fractures, and skeletal deformities during the growth process are common (bossing of skull and malocclusion)

2. Assessment
   a. Note hemoglobin of 5 to 9
   b. Observe for bronze skin
   c. Assess for bone problems and skeletal deformities as described above
   d. Assess for splenomegaly and hepatomegaly
   e. Note possible cardiac involvement from hemosiderosis
3. Interventions
   a. Prepare for and administer multiple blood transfusions
   b. Administer chelating agents to remove excess iron from the system
   c. Prepare for possible splenectomy

G. Sickle-cell anemia

1. Introduction
   a. Autosomal recessive hemolytic anemia; most commonly seen among black Americans
   b. Defective hemoglobin changes the oxygen-carrying capacity and shape of RBCs; altered Hb is referred to as HbS
   c. More than 50% HbS indicates sickle-cell disease; less than 50% HbS indicates sickle-cell trait
   d. RBCs with HbS live less than 20 days
   e. Symptoms of sickle-cell anemia rarely appear before age 4 months because of the predominance of HbF; HbF prevents excessive sickling
   f. Sickle-cell crisis: occurs from dehydration, deoxygenation, or acidosis; changes the RBC to a crescent shape; these altered cells agglutinate; results in occlusion/infarction/ischemia of some body part or organ; infarctions are not caused by a hyperactive clotting mechanism, and anticoagulants are not helpful
   g. Collateral circulation may develop to compensate for prolonged decreased blood supply to an area
2. Assessment: infant
   a. Note colic resulting from pain from an abdominal infarction
   b. Observe for dactylitis/hand-foot syndrome from infarction of short bones
   c. Assess for splenomegaly from sequestered RBCs related to phagocytic function of spleen
3. Assessment: toddler and preschooler
   a. Note hemoglobin of 6 to 9
   b. Assess for hypovolemia and shock from splenic sequestration of large amounts of RBCs
   c. Check for pain at site of vaso-occlusive crisis
4. Assessment: school-age children and adolescents
   a. Review history for pneumococcal pneumonia and other infections from atrophied spleen
   b. Assess for delayed growth and development and delayed sexual maturity
   c. Note and review history for poor wound healing on legs from poor circulation of oxygenated blood to periphery
   d. Ask about priapism and enuresis, common in sickle-cell anemia

5. Interventions to reverse sickling process and promote comfort
   a. Give large amounts of oral or I.V. fluids
   b. Administer oxygen, remove clothing that impedes circulation, reduce energy expenditure to improve oxygenation
   c. Administer pain medication
   d. Provide good skin care and administer antibiotics to prevent infections
   e. Treat acidosis: avoid aspirin because it enhances acidosis and promotes sickling
   f. Maintain normal body temperature in extremities
   g. Implement relaxation techniques to decrease stress
6. Additional nursing interventions
   a. Initiate genetic counseling
   b. Suggest family screening for possible carriers of disease
   c. Teach child to avoid activities that promote crisis

H. Altered clotting function

1. Normal platelet (thrombocyte) function
   a. Platelets are smallest blood element; not nucleated; live 4 to 10 days
   b. They cause capillary homeostasis by adhering to inner surface of vessel and sticking to each other; produce a temporary mechanical plug
   c. They repair breaks in small blood vessels and capillaries, especially in skin, mucous membranes, and internal organs
   d. Interference in platelet function occurs with heparin, aspirin, guaifenesin (Robitussin), indomethacin (Indocin), phenylbutazone (Butazolidin)
2. Normal clotting mechanism
   a. Intrinsic pathway: platelet factor plus antihemophilic factor (Factor VIII) plus multiple clotting factors (including calcium) result in thromboplastin formation; generation of thromboplastin is measured by partial thromboplastin time (PTT)
   b. Extrinsic pathway: injured tissue cells release incomplete thromboplastin; this plus multiple clotting factors results in thromboplastin formation
   c. Prothrombin plus vitamin K (with the help of thromboplastin) result in thrombin production; measured by prothrombin time (PT)
   d. Fibrinogen plus thrombin and Factor VIII result in a fibrin clot; measured by thrombin time

I. Idiopathic thrombocytopenic purpura

1. Introduction
   a. Acquired hemorrhagic disorder resulting in autoimmune destruction of platelets in the spleen
   b. Frequently preceded by an upper respiratory infection or other viral illness
2. Assessment
   a. Assess for petechial rash
   b. Note any bruising or bleeding into urine or stool from low platelet count

3. Interventions
   a. Safety measures to prevent trauma
   b. Prepare for possible splenectomy
   c. Give cortisone or chemotherapeutic drugs to stop the autoimmune process
   d. Administer platelet transfusions
   e. Avoid medicating by injections; if injection is necessary, give subcutaneously and hold pressure on site for 5 minutes
   f. Avoid any aspirin, which will increase bleeding

J. Hemophilia
   1. Introduction
      a. A group of disorders resulting from a deficiency in one of the clotting factors; not a platelet deficiency
      b. Most common types: hemophilia A (Factor VIII deficiency/classical hemophilia), hemophilia B (Factor IX deficiency/Christmas disease), and hemophilia C (Factor XI deficiency)
      c. Hemophilia A involves 75% of all cases; sex-linked recessive disorder
   2. Assessment
      a. Note prolonged bleeding after circumcision, immunizations, or minor injuries
      b. Assess for multiple bruises without petechiae
      c. Check for peripheral neuropathies from bleeding near peripheral nerves
      d. Note elevated PTT
      e. Assess for bleeding into neck, mouth, and thorax, which can seriously threaten respiratory status
      f. Assess for bleeding into a joint (hemarthrosis): measure joint circumference and compare to unaffected joint; note any swelling, pain, limited joint mobility
      g. Assess for any joint degeneration from repeated hemarthroses
   3. Interventions to prevent bleeding
      a. Pad child's environment and toys
      b. Teach parents and child to use protective headgear
      c. Teach parents and child to use soft toothettes instead of bristle toothbrushes
      d. Tell parents to keep weight to low-normal to ease load on joints
      e. Suggest using of stool softeners
      f. Tell child to avoid contact sports
      g. Give cryoprecipitate (frozen Factor VIII) to keep serum level of clotting factor acceptable
      h. Initiate genetic counseling: for male hemophiliac with nonhemophiliac wife, all daughters will be carriers; however, sons will not have the disease; if mother is a carrier and father is a nonhemophiliac, there is a 50% chance with each pregnancy for sons to get hemophilia and a 50% chance for daughters to be carriers

4. Interventions during a bleeding episode
    a. Promote vasoconstriction by applying ice compresses and pressure
    b. Elevate affected extremity above heart
    c. Immobilize site to prevent clots from dislodging
    d. Decrease anxiety to lower child's heart rate
    e. Avoid aspirin, sutures, and cauterization, which may aggravate bleeding
    f. Apply hemostatic agents, such as fibrin foam or topical adrenalin/epinephrine, to promote vasoconstriction
5. Interventions for hemarthrosis
    a. Immobilize affected extremity
    b. Elevate affected extremity in slightly flexed position
    c. Decrease pain and anxiety since these increase heart rate and blood loss
    d. Avoid excessive handling or weight-bearing for 48 hours
    e. Begin mild range-of-motion exercises after 48 hours to facilitate absorption and prevent contractures

Points to Remember

Blood consists of plasma (water, electrolytes, antibodies, clotting factors, proteins) and blood cells (red cells, white cells, and platelets).

Anemias in children are due to alterations in the hemoglobin component, bleeding conditions, hemolysis, or poor iron intake.

Bleeding problems can be caused by platelet dysfunction, deficiency in one of the clotting factors, or bone marrow suppression.

Glossary

Anemia—a decrease in the number or quality of circulating RBCs due to hemorrhage, hemolysis, or lack of production

Hemarthrosis—bleeding into a joint

Polycythemia—overproduction of RBCs, resulting in increased blood viscosity and hematocrit

Altered Immunologic Functioning

Learning Objectives

After studying this section, the reader should be able to:

● Relate allergy and autoimmune disease to abnormal immune function.

● Describe the different types of allergy and plan nursing interventions for Type I allergy.

V. Altered Immunologic Functioning

A. **Alterations in white blood cell (WBC) formation/immune functioning**
1. HLA (human leukocyte antigen/major histocompatibility complex)
   a. Normally found on cell surface of every nucleated cell (not on red blood cells)
   b. Allows body to recognize self versus non-self
   c. Genetically passed on chromosome 6, so child gets markers from both parents
   d. Contains genetic predisposition/susceptibility to disorders; does not pass the disorder itself
   e. Consists of four main loci (HLA-A, HLA-B, HLA-C, HLA-D, HLA-DR)
   f. Likelihood for two people to have same HLA is 1:30,000
   g. For organ transplants, markers matched as closely as possible to decrease possibility of rejection; cornea is avascular and, thus, doesn't need HLA matching
2. Immune system functions
   a. Defense against non-self antigens (hyperfunctioning results in allergy; hypofunction results in immunodeficiency)
   b. Homeostasis; phagocytosis of debris from cellular warfare or of dead cells (hyperfunctioning results in autoimmune disease)
   c. Surveillance/continual alertness to any antigenic invasion (hypofunction results in cancer)
3. Natural first line of defense against disease invasion
   a. Skin
   b. Body secretions (tears, saliva, sebum, mucus, acid environments, normal body flora, salt in sweat)
   c. Nasal hairs and cilia
   d. Controlled temperature
   e. Good renal function
4. Immune cells and their functions
   a. Neutrophil (polymorphonuclear leukocyte): phagocyte; first immune cell at site of trauma; short-lived; attacks bacteria and fungi; bands are immature cells and segmented neutrophils (segs) are mature cells
   b. Eosinophil: effective in phagocytizing parasites; also inactivates histamine and increases with allergic attack
   c. Basophil: releases histamine, SRS-A, and heparin during allergic attack; responsible for many symptoms of anaphylaxis; known as mast cells in tissues
   d. Monocyte: phagocytizes antigens and presents antigenic markers to lymphocytes; appears later than neutrophils but lasts longer; includes Kupffer's cells of liver; macrophage is a monocyte that has left the circulation and entered the tissues

e. B lymphocyte (B cell): produces antibodies; IgM is largest immunoglobulin (Ig), stays in blood, activates complement, is responsible for making antibodies against the ABO blood groups; IgG is smallest Ig and only one that passes placenta, thus offering newborn passive protection, activates complement, has excellent memory; IgD is lymphocyte receptor whose action is not well understood; secretory IgA is present in all moist body secretions, including breast milk, saliva, and tears, prevents adhesion to mucous membranes by virus and bacteria; IgE governs the allergic response by stimulating basophils to release their products after contact with the allergen

f. T lymphocyte (T cell): carries out functions directly or by its cell products; Th (helper T) tells B cells when and how much antibody to make; Ts (suppressor T) tells B cells to stop making antibodies; Te (effector T) mediates multiple immune functions by producing soluble factors (lymphokines); Tc (cytotoxic T) has a direct killing effect

g. Immune cells function in the inflammatory reaction: involves vasodilation (by histamine and SRS-A) and attraction of granulocytes and monocytes to site; cells leave blood and enter damage site, resulting in redness (rubor), warmth (calor), swelling (tumor), and pain (dolor)

B. The febrile child
1. Introduction
   a. Fever is a normal body response to assist the immune system in destroying foreign antigens
   b. Treating fever may mask other signs that would help diagnosis of overtreatment
   c. Temperatures of less than 100° F. (37.8° C.) orally or 100.5° F. (38° C.) rectally normally do not require treatment
2. Interventions
   a. Provide comfort and institute antipyretic actions for temperatures greater than 101.3° F. (38.5° C.)
   b. Give child acetaminophen
   c. Dress child in light pajamas and place in a cool room; cover with sheet only (unless child has chills)
   d. Provide cool fluids and cool, moist compresses to the skin; tepid sponge baths or hypothermia blankets are recommended only for temperatures greater than 104° F. (40° C.), and alcohol baths are not recommended for children
   e. Avoid exposing or cooling child to point of shivering because this will increase body temperature

C. Hypogammaglobulinemia
1. Introduction
   a. Absent or deficient production of B cells; absent or decreased antibody production; may be congenital or acquired

    b. Passive IgG protection from mother to child decreases during first year of life; symptoms usually appear after age 6 months

    c. Patient susceptible to pyogenic bacterial infections

  2. Assessment

    a. Review history for recurrent upper respiratory tract infections, otitis media, skin infections, meningitis, or pneumonia, which are common in hypogammaglobulinemia

    b. Assess for signs and symptoms of malabsorption, which may indicate immunodeficiency

  3. Intervention: give monthly gamma globulin injections

D. Mononucleosis

  1. Introduction

    a. Self-limiting viral infection spread among monocytes

    b. Causative agent: Epstein-Barr virus

    c. Transmission by direct contact of oropharyngeal secretions

    d. Incubation period: 2 to 6 weeks

    e. Prevalent among adolescents

  2. Assessment

    a. Note that complete blood count (CBC) shows atypical monocytes

    b. Note positive Monospot test

    c. Assess for splenomegaly, hepatomegaly, and possible enlargement of lymph nodes

    d. Ask about sore throat and lethargy

  3. Interventions: Provide symptomatic treatment, including increased rest

E. Neutropenia

  1. Introduction

    a. Involves low production of or increased destruction of neutrophils

    b. Results in increased susceptibility to opportunistic infections from the body's inability to initiate the inflammatory response

  2. Assessment

    a. Be aware that signs of inflammation may be altered (no pus, limited redness and swelling)

    b. Assess for irritability, anorexia, and hypothermia, which may be the only symptoms

    c. Note that white blood cell (WBC) count indicates a low absolute neutrophil count (ANC)

  3. Interventions

    a. Decrease contact with pathogens (private room or roommate without infectious process, good handwashing)

    b. Initiate reverse (protective) isolation if ANC less than 500/cu mm

    c. Swab all body orifices frequently to ensure prevention of bacterial growth

    d. Provide good oral hygiene

F. Acquired immune deficiency syndrome (AIDS)
1. Introduction
   a. Acquired immune deficiency from HIV (human immunodeficiency virus) attacking helper T cells
   b. All children in the United States with AIDS are either children of high-risk parents or children who received the virus via blood products
2. Assessment
   a. Check for mononucleosis-like prodromal symptoms
   b. Ask about night sweats
   c. Observe for weight loss and failure to thrive
   d. Assess for lymphadenopathy
   e. Note the presence of recurrent opportunistic infections (especially *Pneumocystis carinii* pneumonia), autoimmune disorders, and malignant neoplasms (especially Kaposi's sarcoma), which are common in AIDS
3. Interventions
   a. Use gloves when changing diapers and when handling body secretions
   b. Practice good handwashing technique
   c. Teach safe sex to adolescents
   d. Use 10% solution of household bleach in water, applied over 1 minute, to kill HIV outside the body

G. Hypersensitivity reactions: Allergy
1. Introduction
   a. Activation of the immune response by normal environmental antigens
   b. Common allergens include inhalants, dust, insect bites, contactants, foods, animal dander, heat, and cold
   c. Exclusively breast-fed infants have a decreased incidence of allergy
   d. Allergic reactions can be immediate or delayed, genetic or acquired
   e. Allergy shots (desensitization) consist of doses of an allergen at levels low enough so that the body does *not* respond; weekly shots of increasing doses can build tolerance; not all allergies can be treated in this way
2. Classification of allergies
   a. Type I (immediate hypersensitivity): IgE-mediated response against allergen; IgE attaches to mast cell, causing it to release histamine; can result in anaphylaxis; is the most common type (examples: hay fever, respiratory allergies, bee stings)
   b. Type II (cytolytic/cytotoxic): antigen is blood-cell bound, resulting in IgM and IgG activating complement (examples: transfusion reactions, Rh incompatibility, idiopathic thrombocytopenic purpura, autoimmune hemolytic anemia)
   c. Type III (immune complex/Arthus reaction): antigen circulates freely, resulting in IgG and IgM response and complement damage of body organs (examples: systemic lupus erythematosus, rheumatic fever, glomerulonephritis, rheumatoid arthritis)

    d. Type IV (delayed hypersensitivity): T cell/cell-mediated; no immunoglobulins are involved; reaction occurs in 48 to 72 hours (examples: contact dermatitis/poison ivy, reactions to tine test, graft rejection)

H. Respiratory allergies
1. Introduction
   a. Type I allergies that release histamine into the eyes, ears, nose, and throat, resulting in discomfort
   b. Occur most often in reaction to inhalants (pollen, animal dander, dust) and injectants (bee stings)
   c. Anaphylaxis can occur with ingestants
2. Assessment
   a. Obtain history of allergies, and how and when symptoms occur
   b. Conduct allergy skin tests to identify cause
   c. Note profuse rhinorrhea
   d. Note allergic shiners (dark circles under eyes from edema)
   e. Note allergic salute (pushing up and out on base of nose)
   f. Check for the crease across bridge of nose from allergic salute
   g. Note open-mouth breathing leading to dry mouth and increasing the risk of respiratory infections
   h. Check for gingival hyperplasia, malocclusion
   i. Note itchy, watery eyes; itching in the back of throat
3. Interventions to relieve attacks
   a. Administer antihistamines
   b. Apply cool compresses to eyes
   c. Administer vasoconstricting nasal sprays
4. Interventions to prevent attacks
   a. Use environmental controls (avoid allergen, keep in air-conditioned room during grass cutting or high pollen count)
   b. Permit only damp dusting
   c. Restrict rugs, stuffed animals, drapes, or natural fibers; use plastic-wrapped mattress
   d. Avoid smoking in child's environment
   e. Administer allergy shots, if appropriate

I. Gastrointestinal allergies
1. Introduction
   a. Allergens include cow's milk, shellfish, nuts, wheat, citrus, berries, egg whites, chocolate, and pork
   b. Food allergy differs from food intolerance conditions, such as celiac disease, PKU, and Crohn's disease
2. Assessment
   a. Review history for types and amounts of food that cause symptoms
   b. Ask how soon symptoms occur after ingestion
   c. Ask what symptoms occur (vomiting, diarrhea, colic, oral skin irritation)
   d. Observe for any failure to thrive

3. Interventions
   a. Identify cause, and eliminate from diet
   b. Feed suspected food again after symptoms disappear, to see if symptoms reappear, unless initial reaction caused anaphylaxis
   c. Be aware that skin tests and allergy shots have not proven beneficial

J. Dermatologic allergies: Eczema

1. Introduction
   a. Type I reaction commonly seen in infants; chronic with exacerbations and remissions
   b. Caused or aggravated by foods, contactants (especially wool), temperature changes, emotional factors, frequent bathing, sweating
2. Assessment
   a. Observe for red, oozing, highly pruritic vesicles that crust
   b. Assess for secondary infections and thickening of the skin from scratching lesions
   c. Check cheeks, scalp, wrists, ankles, and antecubital and popliteal areas, common areas for lesions
   d. Assess for irritability, fretfulness, and insomnia
   e. Observe for dry and scaly skin; hard skin can't trap water
3. Interventions
   a. Use elimination diet to identify cause
   b. Avoid wool; use lightweight cotton
   c. Avoid heat and sweating; keep dry
   d. Give bath only twice per week, without soap if possible
   e. Use Alpha-Keri lotion, and apply topical emollient to skin immediately after bath; pat dry
   f. Keep nails short
   g. Rinse laundry thoroughly, and use mild detergent
   h. Apply cortisone cream to decrease inflammation
   i. Use antipyretics
   j. Use topical lubricating creams on top of hydrocortisone cream
   k. Apply wet compresses with saline or Burow's solution to decrease itching
4. Elimination diet
   a. Eliminate all foods from child's diet except formula
   b. Symptoms should disappear; after 3 days start one food type
   c. Every 3 days, add another food type until symptoms recur or until all foods are resumed
   d. Once offending food is identified, remove it and try it again later after symptoms disappear

Points to Remember

The immune response differentiates self from non-self; alterations in white blood cell function can cause immunodeficiency, allergy, and autoimmune disease.

Allergic reactions can be immediate or delayed, genetic or acquired.

Type I allergy, an IgE-mediated response, is the most common allergic reaction.

Fever is a normal body response to assist the immune system in destroying foreign antigens.

Glossary

Allergic salute—pushing up and out on base of nose to relieve stuffiness

Allergic shiners—dark circles under eyes due to edema and congestion related to histamine

Allergy—hypersensitivity to normal environmental antigens

Human leukocyte antigens (HLAs)—genetically transferred antigenic markers on the cell surface of all nucleated cells that allow the body to recognize self and non-self

Altered CNS Functioning

Learning Objectives

After studying this section, the reader should be able to:

• Describe alterations in the sensory, integrative, and motor functions of the CNS.

• Plan interventions to promote the growth and development, as well as the safety and comfort, of children who have alterations in any component of the sensory motor arc.

• Differentiate among the multiple disorders that can increase intracranial pressure.

VI. Altered CNS Functioning

A. Basic concepts

1. The CNS is a system of communication that receives sensory stimuli from the external (exteroceptors) or internal (interoceptors/proprioceptors) environment; it integrates, perceives, interprets, and/or retains stimuli in memory; stimulus often results in a motor response
2. Senses include vision, hearing, touch, taste, and smell
3. Defects in any phase of the CNS can alter sensory, integrative, and/or motor function; the degree of disability depends on the amount and location of damage
4. Damaged nerve cells cannot be replaced
5. The later a part of the nervous system develops in embryonic life, the more susceptible it is to injury
6. Early infant responses are primarily reflexive; the infant learns to discriminate stimuli and bring motor responses under conscious control
7. Language helps older children improve and increase perception
8. Overload or deprivation of stimuli results in altered CNS functioning

B. Blindness

1. Introduction
   a. Vision provides a spatial sense and has symbolic value
   b. Blind children have no visual memories; they cannot see perspective or reflection and are less motivated to explore
   c. Newborn fixates on light; binocular vision develops at age 4 months
   d. Vision matures at age 6; can use Snellen letter chart after vision matures
2. Assessment of vision
   a. Observe child face to face; eyes should be at same level; juncture of pinna will form a straight line from the lateral corner of the eye
   b. Assess visual acuity using the Snellen symbol chart (ages 3 to 6) or the Snellen letter chart (over age 6)
   c. Check for strabismus
   d. Check for nystagmus
3. Assessment for altered vision
   a. Evaluate growth and development status; child may be slow in acquiring behavior patterns; he may appear delayed in posture control and in acquiring developmental tasks
   b. Observe child's behavior; child may be at a disadvantage in unfamiliar surroundings; he may temporarily be more dependent than usual; he may have frightening experiences, such as feeling that he is falling, which may intimidate him and inhibit exploration
   c. Observe for self-stimulating behaviors, such as eye rubbing or body rocking, which may develop in children with altered vision
   d. Assess child's ability to fixate on objects, to follow a moving light, or to reach out to objects
   e. Note that child will not initiate eye contact with caretaker

    f. Observe for head tilt or frequent blinking or squinting

    g. Ask parent if child holds head very close to books or work

    h. Ask parent if child walks or crawls into furniture or people

4. Interventions

    a. Assist child with understanding of world through other senses

    b. Encourage parents to treat child normally, and encourage stimulation of other senses via play and touch

    c. Encourage exploration and independence; arrange furniture to promote mobility and safety

    d. Act as child's safety advocate

    e. Announce self as you enter room, and explain what you intend to do before doing it

    f. Explain strange sounds

    g. Teach parents tips for children with partial sight: sit child at front of classroom, use large-print materials, use contrasting colors on walls

C. Amblyopia (lazy eye)

1. Introduction

    a. Can result from strabismus

    b. Can cause loss of vision in that eye through disuse

2. Assessment

    a. Note decreased visual acuity in affected eye despite optical correction

    b. Assess for central vision loss of suppressed eye

3. Interventions

    a. Patch healthy eye

    b. Refer for treatment before child is school-age for best results

D. Impaired hearing

1. Introduction

    a. Infant should turn head to locate sound; hearing is fully developed at birth

    b. The ability to hear determines communication, speech, and intellectual functioning

    c. Alterations in the location or shape of ears warrant evaluation of kidney function, since these organs develop simultaneously in utero

    d. Hearing loss is either conductive (middle ear) or sensorineural (inner ear or 8th cranial nerve), caused by infection/inflammation, pressure, or noise

    e. The accumulation of cerumen decreases auditory acuity

2. Assessment

    a. Note if child does not react to or turn to locate sound; does not respond to the repeated calling of his name unless speaker's lips are visible

    b. Note if child does not respond to simple verbal commands or questions; is not soothed by music or by being read to

    c. Assess speech development; child does not develop recognizable speech; either fails to vocalize or remains at the babbling stage

      d. Review history for poor academic performance, using high volumes on radio and TV, straining to hear, or by some speech difficulty, which may indicate mild hearing loss

3. Interventions
   a. Be aware that conductive hearing loss may be remedied by a hearing aid
   b. Encourage face-to-face communication to develop lipreading
   c. Speak clearly and distinctly, but do not exaggerate the pronunciation of words; do not shout; interact in a well-lit environment
   d. Promote communication via sign language and/or verbal communication
   e. Wait for the child's attention before you speak
   f. Use multisensory approaches to develop speech
   g. Promote peer interactions
   h. Use demonstration as a way of explaining before doing treatments

E. Learning disabilities (LD)

1. Introduction
   a. A heterogeneous group of disorders manifested by significant difficulties in listening, speaking, reading, writing, reasoning, or using mathematical abilities; intrinsic to the individual and presumed to be due to CNS dysfunction
   b. Average or above-average IQs present in all children with LD
   c. Affects learning and adapting to life situations; not an academic problem only
   d. Also referred to as an attention deficit disorder

2. Assessment
   a. Assess for *receptive* signs: difficulty remembering the meaning of written symbols; difficulty understanding directions or the tone of conversation; difficulty interpreting body cues, such as the need to defecate or the beginning of menses
   b. Assess for *integrative* signs: difficulty understanding clichés; highly distractable; may see parts but not the whole picture; low information scores on psychological tests; poor reading comprehension
   c. Assess for *motor* signs: poor handwriting; poor hand-eye coordination; hyperactive behavior; reverses letters
   d. Assess for *general* signs: decreased flexibility and ability to adjust; poor school performance despite trying; poor self-esteem related to multiple failures; decreased participation in hobbies/extracurricular activities; decreased curiosity early in life; altered judgment

3. Interventions
   a. Determine most appropriate teaching method for each child; acknowledge the problem, and develop compensatory strategies
   b. Reduce distractions; reduce extraneous information presented; teach in small groups
   c. Understand that a hospital is largely an auditory environment; counteract by writing (printing) information *with* the child
   d. Elicit frequent feedback

e. Repeat directions as often as needed, from the beginning; give a short list of tasks
f. Be aware that a child may have difficulty expressing thoughts, listen to context and give child time to talk; say, "Is this what you mean?"
g. Build on the child's strengths; build self-esteem
h. Introduce parents to the Education for All Handicapped Children Act (PL 94-142), and support their right to have their child tested and educated

F. Hyperactivity (hyperkinetic behavior)
1. Introduction
   a. 25% of children with LD are hyperactive
   b. Behavior may result from a deficit in neurotransmitters
   c. Lasts at least 6 months and is unrelated to psychiatric disorders
2. Assessment
   a. Ask parents if child has increased purposeless physical activity
   b. Assess for decreased attention span
   c. Check for inability to focus attention
   d. Note if child is easily distracted; impulsive
3. Interventions
   a. Administer amphetamines (methylphenidate [Ritalin] or dextroamphetamine [Dexedrine]) to help child concentrate
   b. Provide good patient teaching
   c. Understand that diet control results in controversial and inconsistent results

G. Mental retardation (MR)
1. Introduction
   a. Significantly subaverage general intellectual functioning that exists concurrently with deficits in adaptive behavior and is manifested during the developmental period
   b. Degrees of mental retardation
      Mild: IQ 54 to 69; includes 80% of those labeled MR; educable to 3rd, 4th, or 5th grade level; capable of most independent activities of daily living
      Moderate: IQ 36 to 53; includes 15% of those labeled MR, including most of those with Down's syndrome; trainable self-care to first grade level (mental age 6)
      Severely and profoundly impaired: IQ less than 36; no academic skills; very little independent behavior; cannot protect self; requires complete custodial care
2. Assessment
   a. Assess physical growth parameters and developmental tasks
   b. Assess psychosocial parameters
   c. Make cognitive assessment to determine mental age
   d. Use multiple testing modalities to avoid making an assessment based on a test inappropriate to child's strengths

       e. Arrange at least two testing sessions (a determination of MR is made over time)

       f. Determine family genetics as well as home environment

       g. Compare findings to child's chronologic age

  3. Interventions

       a. Support family during testing

       b. Help parents mourn the loss of the wished-for child

       c. Set realistic, reachable short-term goals; break tasks into small steps to encourage successful accomplishment

       d. Help parents avoid frustration; achievement will occur slowly

       e. Apply behavior modification, if applicable

       f. Stimulate and communicate at the child's mental rather than chronologic age

       g. Physically stimulate via rocking and bathing

       h. Promote normalization; seek mainstreaming

       i. Act as a safety advocate

H. Cerebral palsy (CP)

  1. Introduction

       a. A neuromuscular disorder resulting from damage to or aberrant structure of the area of the brain that controls motor function

       b. Caused by trauma/hemorrhage or anoxia to areas of brain occurring before birth, perinatally, or postnatally

       c. A nonprogressive disorder; only the complications of CP can progress

  2. Assessment

       a. Assess for signs and symptoms of *spastic* CP: hypertonicity; leg scissoring; persistent primitive reflexes; inadequate protective reflexes; altered quality of speech; poor coordination; persistent muscle contraction, resulting in contractures

       b. Assess for signs and symptoms of *dyskinetic/athetotic* CP: abnormal, constant involuntary wormlike movements that disappear during sleep and increase with stress, especially affects facial muscles; decreased ability in fine motor skills; no contractures

       c. Assess for signs and symptoms of *ataxic* CP: poor equilibrium and muscle coordination; unsteady, wide-based gait

       d. Assess for signs and symptoms of *rigid* CP: simultaneous contraction of contracting and extensor muscles, resulting in resistance to movement, diminished reflexes, and severe contractures

  3. Interventions

       a. Increase caloric intake for athetotic CP because of constant movement

       b. Mash or process food to make it easy to manage; decrease stress during mealtimes

       c. Provide safe environment, such as protective headgear or bed pads

       d. Provide rest periods

       e. Use range-of-motion exercises, if spastic; maintain proper alignment

       f. Promote age-appropriate mental activities and incentives for motor development

    g. Break down tasks into small steps
    h. Refer child for speech, nutrition, and physical therapy
    i. Promote positive self-concept
  4. Disabilities associated with CP
    a. MR of varying degrees (in 18% to 50%); most children with CP have at least a normal IQ but can't demonstrate it on standardized tests
    b. Speech defects
    c. Dental anomalies
    d. Seizures
    e. Vision and/or hearing disturbances
    f. Poor self-image; low self-esteem

I. Seizure disorders

  1. Introduction
    a. Seizure: a sudden episodic, involuntary alteration in consciousness, motor activity, behavior, sensation, or autonomic function; nerve cells become hyperexcitable and surpass the seizure threshold; neurons overfire without regard to stimuli or need
    b. Convulsion: used synonymously with seizure; involuntary muscular contraction and relaxation
    c. Epilepsy: an intermittent disorder of the nervous system resulting in many types of recurrent seizures; produced by excessive neuronal discharges
  2. Assessment
    a. Ask if the child experiences an aura (preictal): peculiar sensations experienced just before seizure onset (unusual tastes, feelings, odors)
    b. Determine nature of the seizure: What muscles are involved? How are they positioned? Is there symmetry of movement? What is level of consciousness? What is patient's respiratory status? Is patient continent or incontinent?
    c. Determine postictal response: Is patient oriented to time and place? Is patient drowsy and uncoordinated?
    d. Note altered electroencephalogram (EEG)
  3. Interventions
    a. Stay with child
    b. Move child to flat surface, out of danger
    c. Provide patent airway; place child on side to let saliva drain out
    d. Do not try to interrupt the seizure
    e. Gently support head and keep hands from hurting self, but *do not restrain*
    f. *Do not use tongue depressors;* they add stimuli
    g. Reduce external stimuli
    h. Loosen tight clothing
    i. Record seizure activity
    j. Pad crib or bed

CLASSIFICATION OF SEIZURES

TYPE	DESCRIPTION	SYMPTOMS
I Partial	Localized to one area of brain (but may progress to generalized)	
A. Simple partial	Symptoms confined to one hemisphere	May have motor (change in posture), sensory (hallucinations), or autonomic (flushing, tachycardia) symptoms; no loss of consciousness
B. Complex partial	Begins in one focal area but spreads to both hemispheres (more common in adults)	Loss of consciousness; aura of visual disturbances; postictal symptoms
II Generalized	Initial onset occurs in both hemispheres	Loss of consciousness; bilateral motor activity
A. Absence (petit mal)	Sudden onset; lasts 5 to 10 seconds; can have 100 daily; precipitated by stress, hyperventilation, hypoglycemia, fatigue; differentiated from daydreaming	Loss of responsiveness but continued ability to maintain posture control and not fall; twitching eyelids; lip smacking; no postictal symptoms
B. Myoclonic	Movement disorder (not a seizure); seen as child awakens or falls asleep; may be precipitated by touch or visual stimuli; focal or generalized; symmetrical or asymmetrical	No loss of consciousness; sudden, brief shocklike involuntary contraction of one muscle group
C. Infantile spasms	Jitteriness of a muscle group	Flexed trunk; drawn-up legs; extended arms; nodding of head momentarily; laughter or crying may accompany attack
D. Clonic	Opposing muscles contract and relax alternately in rhythmic pattern; may occur in one limb more than others	Mucus production
E. Tonic	Muscles are maintained in continuous contracted state (rigid posture)	Variable loss of consciousness; pupils dilate; eyes roll up; glottis closes; possible incontinence; may foam at mouth
F. Tonic-clonic (grand mal/ major motor)	Violent total body seizure	Aura; tonic first (20 to 40 seconds); clonic next; postictal symptoms
G. Atonic	Drop and fall attack; needs to wear protective helmet	Loss of posture tone
H. Akinetic	Sudden brief loss of muscle tone or posture	Temporary loss of consciousness
III Miscellaneous A. Febrile	Seizure threshold lowered by elevated temperature; only one seizure per fever; common in 5% of population under age 5; occurs when temperature is rapidly rising	Lasts less than 5 minutes; generalized, transient and nonprogressive; does not generally result in brain damage; EEG is normal after 2 weeks
B. Status epilepticus	Prolonged or frequent repetition of seizures without interruption; results in anoxia, cardiac and respiratory arrest	Patient does not regain consciousness between seizures; lasts more than 30 minutes

k. Administer phenytoin (Dilantin) to decrease neuron excitability and to keep it below the seizure threshold. Side effects include gum hyperplasia, hirsutism, ataxia, gastric distress, nystagmus, anemia, and sedation.

l. Administer phenobarbital to increase seizure threshold and inhibit spread of electrical discharge; often given with Dilantin because of its potentiating effect

m. Provide a ketogenic (high-fat) diet: ketones develop through fasting and are thought to raise the seizure threshold

J. Increased intracranial pressure (ICP)

1. Introduction
   a. May be caused by inflammatory process, tissue enlargement, increased fluid accumulation
   b. Swelling results in pressure on brain tissue with altered brain function
2. Assessment of child after closure of cranial sutures
   a. Check for nausea and/or vomiting
   b. Check for headache
   c. Take vital signs; note increased blood pressure, decreased pulse rate, and decreased respiratory rate
   d. Assess for blurred vision, papilledema, altered pupillary reaction to light
   e. Personality changes
   f. Observe and monitor seizures
   g. Assess for altered level of consciousness with decreased attention span and/or lethargy
   h. Observe for alteration in motor skills; appears clumsy, loses balance
   i. Monitor for altered vital signs; can deteriorate to respiratory and cardiac arrest
3. Assessment of child before closure of cranial sutures (See "Hydrocephalus")
4. Interventions
   a. Elevate head of bed slightly to decrease cerebral edema
   b. Administer osmotic diuretics (mannitol) to decrease cerebral edema
   c. Administer corticosteroids to decrease brain inflammation
   d. Limit fluids to decrease blood volume, which will decrease cerebral edema
   e. Monitor fluid and electrolytes
   f. Perform hyperventilation with a bag-valve-mask device
   g. Monitor level of consciousness

K. Hydrocephalus

1. Introduction
   a. An increase in the amount of cerebrospinal fluid (CSF) in ventricles and subarachnoid spaces of brain
   b. Overproduction of CSF by choroid plexus
   c. Noncommunicating hydrocephalus: blockage of flow of CSF from tumors, hemorrhage, or structural abnormalities, resulting in fluid accumulation in ventricles

     d. Communicating hydrocephalus: abnormal absorption of CSF after it reaches subarachnoid space due to scarring, congenital anomalies, or hemorrhage; there is no blockage of fluid

  2. Assessment of child before closure of cranial sutures
     a. Measure head circumference; note rapid increase
     b. Observe for full, tense, bulging fontanels
     c. Check for widening of suture lines
     d. Observe for distended scalp veins
     e. Assess for irritability or lethargy; decreased attention span
     f. Note high-pitched cry
     g. Note sunset sign (sclera visible above iris)
     h. Observe for inability to support head when upright
     i. Percuss skull; note "cracked pot" sound
     j. Perform transillumination of skull; light will reflect off opposite side of skull

  3. Interventions: shunt insertion
     a. Assist doctor as he threads thin shunt tubing with a one-way valve, from lateral ventricle, behind ear and down neck and chest, to peritoneum or right atrium
     b. *Do not* lay child on side of body where shunt is located after shunt insertion
     c. Elevate head of bed slightly
     d. Observe for blockage of shunt with signs of increased ICP
     e. Observe for signs of infection
     f. Be aware that if caudal end of shunt must be externalized because of infection, the bag *must be kept at ear level* to prevent increase or decrease in ICP
     g. Assist doctor as he lengthens shunt tubing as child grows; this process will probably be initiated by blockage of shunt and a resulting increase in ICP
     h. Support head when child is upright
     i. Provide good skin care to head; turn frequently

L. Brain tumors
  1. Introduction
     a. Second most prevalent type of cancer in children
     b. Peak ages for brain tumors at diagnosis are ages 3 to 7
     c. Two thirds of pediatric brain tumors are infratentorial, often involving the cerebellum or brain stem
     d. Gliomas are the most common brain tumors in children
     e. Generally results in a poor prognosis
     f. Types of brain tumors most commonly seen: medulloblastoma, astrocytoma, ependymoma, glioma, craniopharyngioma

  2. Assessment
     a. Symptoms stem from the tumor's pressure on adjacent neural tissues

    b. Young children are often difficult to diagnose because of the elasticity of their skulls and normally poor coordination

    c. Decrease in school performance may be first sign

    d. Note signs of increased ICP

    e. Alterations in neurologic function, especially visual acuity and behavior changes, may occur

    f. Headache, commonly an initial sign, usually occurs in the early morning

    g. Note vomiting, hypotonia, posturing, seizures, altered vital signs

    h. Assess for signs and symptoms of *medulloblastoma:* ataxia, early-morning vomiting, anorexia

    i. Assess for signs and symptoms of *astrocytoma:* papilledema, blindness

    j. Assess for signs and symptoms of *ependymoma:* increased intracranial pressure (see "Increased intracranial pressure"), difficulty swallowing, paresthesias, abdominal pain, vertigo, head tilt

    k. Assess for signs and symptoms of *glioma:* ataxia, cranial nerve palsies

    l. Assess for signs and symptoms of *craniopharyngioma:* pressure on pituitary, resulting in diabetes insipidus; visual problems; difficulty regulating body temperature; altered growth patterns; altered CSF pressure

3. Interventions (preoperatively)

    a. Prepare child for computed tomography scan or magnetic resonance imaging

    b. Prepare child for facial edema and hair loss

    c. Prepare child for radiation treatments, which may be given to shrink tumor

4. Interventions (postoperatively)

    a. Position on nonoperative site to decrease pressure

    b. Make sure child lies flat on either side if surgery was infratentorial; elevate head of bed slightly if surgery was supratentorial

    c. Monitor vital signs; check pupils

    d. Assess level of consciousness and ease of arousal

    e. Relieve eye edema with cold compresses, lubricate eyes

    f. Prevent increased ICP by preventing straining at stool or forceful coughing

    g. Initiate seizure precautions

    h. Administer vasopressin (Pitressin) to treat diabetes insipidus

M. Myelomeningocele/meningomyelocele/spina bifida

1. Introduction

    a. Posterior portion of laminae of vertebrae fails to close anywhere along the spinal cord

    b. Occurs at 3 to 4 weeks of gestation

    c. Sac includes spinal nerves, causing multiple handicaps

    d. Surgical correction usually occurs within 48 hours of birth

    e. Defect can be detected early in gestation; amniotic fluid will contain high levels of alpha-fetoprotein from leaking CSF

2. Assessment (preoperatively)
    a. Check for leakage from sac
    b. Check for infection around sac
    c. Assess for signs and symptoms of CNS infection
    d. Assess for motor activity below sac
    e. Measure head circumference to get baseline
    f. Assess bowel and bladder function
3. Interventions (preoperatively)
    a. Provide emotional support to parents
    b. Prevent trauma by keeping pressure off sac; keep child on side with knees flexed or on abdomen
    c. Institute measures to keep sac free of infection; avoid contamination from urine and stool
    d. Prevent sac from drying; cover it with saline-soaked sterile dressings
4. Assessment (postoperatively)
    a. Note degree of leg movement in response to discomfort
    b. Note degree of sensitivity to touch below level of lesion; paralysis is possible
    c. Observe for clubfoot
    d. Observe for dribbling of urine or involuntary release of stool, which may indicate neurogenic bladder and bowel
    e. Observe for signs of increased ICP; it may be related to scarring of spinal area from reduced absorptive space
5. Interventions (postoperatively)
    a. Provide routine postoperative care
    b. Perform Credé's maneuver to empty bladder
    c. Provide skin care if paralysis occurs
    d. Provide orthopedic appliances, if necessary
    e. Prevent constipation
    f. Promote independence

N. Meningitis
1. Introduction
    a. Inflammation of meninges
    b. Caused by viral or bacterial agents; transmitted by droplet spread
    c. Organisms enter blood from nasopharynx or middle ear
    d. Most common in infants and toddlers
2. Assessment
    a. Note seizures
    b. Observe for signs of increased ICP: vomiting, irritability, hyperesthesia
    c. Note Brudzinski's sign (child will flex knees and hips in response to passive neck flexion)
    d. Assess for abnormal postures such as opisthotonos
    e. Note Kernig's sign
    f. Check ear drainage for presence of CSF by testing it for glucose; CSF tests positive for glucose

    g. Assess for purpuric rash, which may indicate meningoccal meningitis

    h. Note that lumbar puncture will show increased CSF pressure, cloudy color, increased WBC and protein counts, and decreased glucose count if meningitis caused by bacteria

  3. Interventions

    a. Institute seizure control measures

    b. Isolate for at least 24 hours after antibiotic therapy begins

    c. Assess neurologic status frequently to monitor for increased ICP

    d. Provide dark and quiet environment

    e. Keep child flat in bed

    f. Move child gently

    g. Administer parenteral antibiotics

O. Reye's syndrome

  1. Introduction

    a. An acute encephalopathy with cerebral cortex swelling but without inflammation

    b. Accompanied by impaired liver function and hyperammonemia

    c. Usually preceded by a viral infection and the use of aspirin

  2. Assessment

    a. Assess for signs and symptoms of Stage I: apparent recovery from viral infection, followed suddenly by vomiting, lethargy, drowsiness, and liver dysfunction

    b. Assess for signs and symptoms of Stage II: disorientation, hyperventilation, hyperactive reflexes, hyperammonemia; positive response to noxious stimuli

    c. Assess for signs and symptoms of Stage III: coma, decorticate rigidity, obtundation; equal and reactive pupils

    d. Assess for signs and symptoms of Stage IV: decerebrate posture; unresponsive pupils; apparent liver improvement

    e. Assess for signs and symptoms of Stage V: seizures, loss of deep tendon reflexes (DTR), normal ammonia level, respiratory arrest

  3. Interventions

    a. Expect that child will be cared for in intensive care unit

    b. Monitor and maintain normal body functions and provide comfort measures

    c. Support family

    d. Expect to induce barbiturate coma or administer pancuronium (Pavulon) to paralyze skeletal muscles and prevent further increase of ICP, if necessary in late stages

Points to Remember

The CNS includes sensory, integrative, and motor functions; alterations can occur in any or all of them.

Alterations from blindness or deafness require compensation by other senses.

Alterations anywhere in the CNS require nursing interventions designed to adjust the environment, maintain safety, and promote growth and development.

Neurologic signs must be properly identified so that children with one disability or disease are not labeled incorrectly (for example, LD and CP children should not be labeled mentally retarded simply because they cannot perform certain motor tasks).

Glossary

Astrocytoma (in cerebellum)—benign, slow-growing cysts; symptoms are due to focal pressure of tumor; surgery after early diagnosis results in a high cure rate

Craniopharyngioma (in sella turcica)—the most common nongliomatous brain tumor in children; disturbs endocrine function and vision; presses on third ventricle; arises from remnants of embryonic tissue; surgery has variable results

Ependymoma (in ventricles)—results in noncommunicating hydrocephalus; usually benign but pressure can damage vital organs; surgery is partially successful

Gliomas (in brain stem)—slow-growing tumors; usually inoperable because of location

Medulloblastoma (in cerebellum)—a highly malignant, fast-growing tumor; radiation is used since complete excision is difficult

Neurogenic bladder—dribbling of urine from lack of spontaneous emptying of bladder

Nystagmus—an involuntary rapid, jerky movement of the eye

Strabismus—eyes are misaligned when fixating on the same object, from a muscle imbalance; can be treated by surgery and/or eye exercises

Altered Respiratory Functioning

Learning Objectives

After studying this section, the reader should be able to:

• Assess respiratory distress in a child.

• Describe conditions or complications related to immature lung development in children.

• Explain the treatments most commonly implemented for respiratory conditions.

• Differentiate among various childhood respiratory conditions, and plan appropriate nursing interventions.

VII. Altered Respiratory Functioning

A. Basic concepts

1. Development of the respiratory system
   a. Lungs are not fully developed at birth
   b. Alveoli continue to grow and increase in size through age 8
   c. Infants are obligate nose breathers
   d. Infants are diaphragmatic breathers
   e. Child's respiratory tract has a narrower lumen than an adult's until age 5
   f. Narrow airway makes the young child prone to possible airway inflammation and obstuction, and respiratory distress
   g. Respiratory rate is 60 at birth and decreases with age
2. Respiratory distress results in suprasternal, intercostal, and substernal retractions as other muscles assist with breathing

B. Respiratory distress

1. Assessment
   a. Observe child's face for signs of anxiety
   b. Observe position child maintains to ease respiratory effort (usually sits up or hyperextends neck)
   c. Evaluate energy and effort needed for child to breathe
   d. Assess respiratory quantity and quality: tachypnea (fast respiratory rate), hyperpnea (deep respirations), apnea (unintentional cessation in spontaneous breathing for more than 20 seconds with bradycardia and color change)
   e. Assess symmetry of chest movement
   f. Assess for irritability
   g. Assess for change in chest configuration to accommodate increased air trapping (barrel chest) or for congenital chest deformities that interfere with adequate respiratory effort (pigeon chest, pectus excavatum)
   h. Assess for nasal flaring (nares widen on inhalation)
   i. Assess for open-mouth breathing and chin lag (chin lowers with inhalation)
   j. Assess for skin color change: paleness, cyanosis (especially circumoral cyanosis)
   k. Assess for accessory muscle use: upper neck muscles strain with inhalation (tracheal tugging); lower muscle use (below rib cage)
   l. Assess for retractions: suprasternal (directly above sternum), intercostal (between ribs), substernal (below xiphoid process)
   m. Assess for finger and toe clubbing (proliferation of terminal phalangeal tissue) from hypoxia
   n. Assess cardiac tolerance of respiratory alteration
   o. Measure respiratory capacity using pulmonary function tests (may not effectively measure capacity in young children because they have trouble following directions)
   p. Evaluate chest X-rays (ensure adequate protection by covering gonads and thyroid gland with lead apron)

q. Monitor blood gas measurements
r. Auscultate lungs for absent or diminished breath sounds and inspiratory or expiratory wheeze (whistling noise as air is forced through a narrow passage)
s. Assess for expiratory grunt as lower accessory muscles force air out
t. Assess for inspiratory stridor (harsh sound from laryngeal or tracheal edema)
u. Assess for hoarse cough or muffled speech
v. Assess for cough, and note whether it's dry or congested, productive or nonproductive (a cough is productive if child coughs up and swallows mucus; mucus need not be expectorated for cough to be considered productive), paroxysmal or intermittent

2. Interventions
a. Expect possible use of *oxygen tent;* keep sides of plastic down and tucked in because oxygen is heavier than air, so loss will be greater at bottom of tent; keep plastic away from child's face; prevent use of toys that produce sparks or friction; frequently assess oxygen concentration; to return child to a tent after removing him for any reason, put tent sides down, turn on oxygen, wait until oxygen is at ordered concentration, then place child in tent
b. Expect possible use of *cool mist tents* (croup tents); used to make mucus thin, these tents make expectoration easier; provide same care as with oxygen tent; expect child to be fearful if mist prevents him from seeing environment; encourage use of transitional objects in tent, except for stuffed toys, which may become damp and promote bacterial growth; keep child dry by changing bed linens and pajamas frequently; maintain steady body temperature
c. Teach parents about *cool mist vaporizers* for home use; tell them to clean frequently to prevent germs from being sprayed into the air
d. Perform *chest physiotherapy, percussion, and postural drainage:* loosens secretions and enhances their expectoration via gravity; perform at least 30 minutes before meals; use cupped hand over a covered rib cage for 2 to 5 minutes on each of the five positions; don't do this during acute bronchoconstriction (for example, asthma) or airway edema (for example, croup) to prevent mucus plugs from loosening and causing airway obstruction
e. Administer *aerosol nebulized medications* immediately before percussion and postural drainage
f. Perform *nasal suctioning* using a bulb syringe or nasotracheal suction using low pressure
g. Use *saline solution nose drops* to relieve nasal stuffiness; teach family how to prepare this solution at home by mixing ⅛ teaspoon salt in 4 oz sterile water; administer 1 to 2 drops in each nostril and use bulb suction if needed
h. Teach child *breathing exercises* to enhance aeration and increase respiratory muscle tone; teach exercises to expand chest (deep breathing), to compress chest (sit-ups or toe touching), and to increase respiratory

efficiency (jumping jacks); make each exercise into a game (for example, "Simon says, touch your toes"); do not let child overdo exercises to the point of fatigue

 i. Teach parents how to use *apnea monitors* at home (usually involve the application of three leads); although they help reassure parents, alarm may sound frightening; teach parents how to assess child and machine when alarm sounds

 j. Organize activities to include rest periods; elevate head of bed or use infant seat to take pressure off abdominal organs and diaphragm

 k. Avoid oral feeding if child has tachypnea or dyspnea; if child's in mild distress, encourage small, frequent, slow feeding of clear liquids to prevent aspiration; avoid milk (it tends to promote phlegm production)

 l. Expect to give antihistamines if symptoms stem from allergy; these medications not given for the common cold because they dry up secretions, countering measures aimed at liquefying them

 m. Administer decongestants

 n. Administer antitussives for dry cough; do not try to suppress a productive cough

 o. Teach parents to avoid the use of respiratory irritants, such as baby powder or cigarette smoke

C. Upper respiratory infections/nasopharyngitis

1. Introduction
   a. Only the upper airway is involved
   b. Nasal blockage interferes with feeding since infants are nose breathers
   c. Rhinorrhea may be serous or mucopurulent
   d. A child normally has six to nine colds per year
2. Assessment
   a. Assess degree of respiratory distress
   b. Check temperature
   c. Check throat for white lesions, and take culture if appropriate
   d. Differentiate colds from respiratory allergies by history
   e. Assess change in behavior
3. Interventions
   a. Take measures to reduce fever
   b. Provide decongestants and a vaporizer, and encourage rest and increased fluid intake
   c. Use saline nose drops and bulb syringe on infant
   d. Administer antibiotics if bacterial cause is suspected

D. Tonsillitis

1. Introduction
   a. Tonsils are lymph organs guarding the entrance to the respiratory and gastrointestinal systems
   b. They should not be removed unless they occlude the airway, have atrophied and no longer function, or are chronically infected

      c. Tonsillitis can be treated with antibiotics at home; tonsillectomy requires prehospitalization teaching for a 1-day or overnight procedure

  2. Assessment

      a. Review history for evidence of allergy symptoms

      b. Note symptoms of allergic disorders

      c. Assess for signs of ear infection

      d. Assess respiratory effort

  3. Interventions (preoperative)

      a. Explain why the child is coming to the hospital

      b. Use words like "fix your tonsils" rather than "take out"

      c. Encourage parents to stay with child until surgery

      d. Prepare child for sights and sounds of surgery

      e. Allow child to play with equipment

      f. Assure child that he will never be alone and will not feel the procedure

      g. Call anesthesia "special sleep" instead of "sleeping medicine"

      h. Put transitional object in recovery room for child

      i. Prepare child for a sore throat

      j. Inspect mouth for loose teeth; evaluate for signs and symptoms of upper respiratory infection

  4. Interventions (postoperative)

      a. Place child in prone or side-lying position to facilitate drainage

      b. Do not suction unless there is an obstruction, this will decrease trauma to site

      c. Check for frequent swallowing; restlessness; fast, thready pulse; and/or vomiting bright red blood; they are signs of hemorrhage and require immediate attention; vomiting dried blood is common

      d. Provide ice collar for comfort and for reducing edema

      e. Provide clear, cool, noncitrus, nonred fluids

      f. Engage child in therapeutic doll play to help him deal with his feelings and confusion about the procedure after he recovers

E. Epiglottitis

  1. Introduction

      a. A potentially life-threatening infection of the epiglottis

      b. Preschool age-group (ages 3 to 6) is most commonly affected

      c. *Hemophilus influenzae* is most common organism

  2. Assessment

      a. Assess for difficult and painful swallowing; note increased drooling, refusal to drink, and stridor

      b. Listen for muffled speech

      c. Note fever, irritability, restlessness

      d. Note rapid pulse rate and respirations; child may extend neck

      e. Ask about sore throat

  3. Interventions

      a. Defer inspecting throat until arrival of emergency personnel and supplies; inspection could stimulate spasm of epiglottis and cause respiratory occlusion

      b. Allow child to sit up; this makes breathing easier

      c. Have equipment ready for tracheotomy or intubation

      d. Administer antibiotics

F. Croup/acute spasmodic laryngitis/acute obstructive laryngitis/acute laryngotracheobronchitis

  1. Introduction

      a. A group of related entities most common among toddlers

      b. Caused by virus-induced edema around the larynx, accompanied by a barking cough

      c. Often begins at night and during cold weather

      d. Recurs often; sudden onset or slowly progressive

  2. Assessment

      a. Note barking, brassy cough; hoarseness

      b. Note inspiratory stridor with varying degrees of respiratory distress

      c. Assess for increased dyspnea and lower accessory muscle use; rales and decreased breath sounds, which may indicate that the condition has progressed to bronchi

  3. Interventions (for the child at home)

      a. Tell parents to keep child calm to ease respiratory effort and conserve energy

      b. Tell parents to take child to bathroom, close door, and turn on shower *hot* water spigot full-force; sit on bathroom floor with child on lap as room fills with steam; this should decrease laryngeal spasm

      c. After an acute episode, use vaporizer near child's bed

      d. After a crisis, mucus production increases, and child may vomit large amounts of it; this vomiting does not require treatment

      e. Encourage clear liquid intake to keep mucus thin

      f. Caution parents that if crisis does not resolve, child may need hospitalization for tracheostomy, oxygen, and mist

G. Otitis media (middle ear infection)

  1. Introduction

      a. Very common in infants since ear canal is shorter and less angled

      b. Often a complication of upper respiratory infections, due to blockage of eustachian tubes (results in unequal pressure between middle ear and outside environment and possible introduction of virus or bacteria into middle ear)

  2. Assessment

      a. Assess for bulging, red tympanic membrane

      b. Assess for pain; note that infant pulls on ear when he has pain

      c. Observe for irritability

      d. Assess for signs and symptoms of upper respiratory infection

      e. Note degree of fever

  3. Interventions (for acute otitis media)

      a. Administer antibiotics orally or as eardrops

    b. Remember to pull earlobe down and back when administering eardrops in infants

    c. Administer analgesics and antipyretics

    d. Administer decongestants to relieve eustachian tube obstruction

4. Interventions (for chronic otitis media)

    a. Be aware that surgery (myringotomy) will be performed to drain middle ear and equalize pressure (tubes inserted at the time of surgery often fall out within 1 year)

    b. Position child on affected side to facilitate drainage if tympanic membrane ruptures or after myringotomy

    c. Keep ear canal clean and dry; keep water out of ears

H. Bronchiolitis caused by respiratory syncytial virus (RSV) infection

1. Introduction

    a. A lower respiratory infection characterized by thick mucus

    b. Infants younger than age 6 months are most commonly affected; winter and spring are most common seasons

    c. RSV infection is the most common cause of bronchiolitis in infants, with a mortality in this population of 1% to 6%

    d. Respiratory secretions spread the disease, not droplets

2. Assessment

    a. Be aware that very thick mucus is possible

    b. Assess for possible air trapping and atelectasis

    c. Suction bronchial aspirate of mucus for testing for RSV to confirm the diagnosis

3. Interventions

    a. Provide humidified oxygen

    b. Expect to give intravenous fluids

    c. Use gloves, gowns, and good handwashing as secretion precautions

I. Asthma

1. Introduction

    a. A reversible, diffuse, obstructive pulmonary disease due to hyperreaction of the lower respiratory tract to an environmental allergen; cause may be idiopathic or intrinsic

    b. Bronchoconstriction from asthma restricts airflow

    c. Asthma results in edema of the mucous membranes, smooth muscle bronchospasm, and an accumulation of tenacious mucus

2. Assessment

    a. Evaluate degree of respiratory distress and dyspnea and use of accessory muscles; note unequal breath sounds

    b. Auscultate for prolonged expiration with presence of expiratory wheeze; in severe distress, inspiratory wheeze may be heard

    c. Review history for exercise intolerance

    d. Note fatigue and apprehension

    e. Observe for diaphoresis

    f. Allow child to sit upright to ease breathing

g. Observe for alteration in contour of chest due to chronic air trapping
h. Ask about positive family history of allergies; positive patient history of eczema or other allergies
i. Evaluate blood gas measurement; may show increased $PaCO_2$ from respiratory acidosis
j. Assess neurologic status; severe hypoxia can alter cerebral function

3. Interventions (to prevent attack)
a. Remove offending allergen; test skin to identify source of allergy; hyposensitization
b. Modify environment to avoid allergic reaction
c. Administer cromolyn sodium, an inhalant; prevents release of mast cell products after antigen-IgE reaction
d. Teach breathing exercises to increase ventilatory capacity

4. Interventions (during acute asthmatic attack)
a. Administer methylxanthines such as theophylline, that act as bronchodilators; monitor for gastrointestinal distress and alteration in vital signs, especially cardiac stimulation and hypotension
b. Give corticosteroids to decrease edema of mucous membranes
c. Provide moist oxygen
d. Administer I.V. fluids
e. Forbid smoking in child's environment
f. Be aware that failure of the child to respond to drugs during an acute attack can result in status asthmaticus

J. Cystic fibrosis (CF)

1. Introduction
a. An inherited autosomal recessive disease of the exocrine glands
b. The most common genetic disease in the United States
c. Death is almost always due to respiratory incompetence
d. 85% of patients have little or no release of pancreatic enzymes (lipase, amylase, and trypsin)
e. Airway is obstructed by increased and constant production of mucus
f. Children with CF sweat normally, but their sweat contains 2 to 5 times the normal levels of sodium and chloride
g. Males are sterile due to blockage or absence of vas deferens; females have increased mucus in their reproductive tract, making conception difficult
h. Portal hypertension related to cirrhosis of the liver can result in esophageal varices
i. Salt depletion may occur during hot weather and heavy exercise

2. Assessment
a. Assess for meconium ileus in newborns from lack of pancreatic enzymes
b. Observe for bulky, greasy, foul-smelling stools that contain undigested food
c. Assess for failure to thrive from malabsorption
d. Observe for distended abdomen and thin arms and legs from steatorrhea

    e. Be aware that child has a voracious appetite from undigested food lost in stool

    f. Conduct pilocarpine iontophoresis sweat test

    g. Check for salty taste on child's skin

    h. Assess for degree of respiratory distress

    i. Review history for chronic, productive cough with frequent *Pseudomonas* infections

    j. Note typical signs of a chronic obstructive respiratory disease

3. Interventions

    a. Administer pancreatic enzymes *with* meals and snacks

    b. Provide high-calorie, high-protein, low-fat foods with added salt

    c. Give multivitamins twice a day, especially if they are fat-soluble vitamins

    d. Perform pulmonary hygiene (chest percussion and postural drainage) two to four times per day, preceded by mucolytic, bronchodilator, and/or antibiotic nebulizer inhalation treatment

    e. Encourage physical activity and/or creative breathing exercises

    f. Teach parents to avoid administering cough suppressants and antihistamines, since the child needs to be able to cough and expectorate

    g. Administer I.V. antibiotics for *Pseudomonas* infection only when the infection interferes with daily functioning

    h. Initiate genetic counseling for the family

    i. Promote as normal a life as possible

K. Respiratory distress syndrome (RDS)

1. Introduction

    a. Hyaline membrane disease is previous name

    b. A disease of prematurity from underdeveloped and uninflated alveoli and the absence of surfactant

2. Assessment

    a. Observe for respiratory distress, grunting respirations, increased respiratory rate

    b. Note that X-ray has ground glass appearance

    c. Note that increased energy is required to breathe, which may result in exhaustion

    d. Note that blood gas measurements are abnormal

3. Interventions

    a. Expect child to be on a ventilator to keep alveoli open; administer oxygen

    b. Organize care to ensure minimal handling

    c. Control temperature to reduce stress and decrease additional energy use

    d. Use aseptic technique to reduce risk of infection

    e. Administer I.V. fluids to ensure good hydration but withhold food and fluids because of high respiratory rate; expect possible nasogastric tube feedings

    f. Turn every 2 hours; raise head of bed; perform chest percussion before suctioning

    g. Enhance bonding between parents and child

L. Bronchopulmonary dysplasia (BPD)
1. Introduction
   a. A complication of RDS resulting from high oxygen concentration and long-term assisted ventilation
   b. Epithelial damage occurs with thickening and fibrotic proliferation of the alveolar walls and damage to the bronchiolar epithelium
   c. Ciliary activity is inhibited so child has trouble clearing mucus from lungs
   d. Recovery usually occurs in 6 to 12 months; however, child may remain ventilator-dependent for years
2. Assessment
   a. Be aware that there may be no symptoms
   b. Monitor chest X-ray results; pulmonary changes may be the only way to diagnose BPD
3. Interventions
   a. Anticipate continued ventilatory support and oxygen
   b. Continue supportive measures to enhance respiratory function
   c. Begin an intensive program to promote normal development
   d. Provide adequate time for rest
   e. Encourage parents to visit and become involved in care since child may require lengthy hospitalization

M. Foreign-body aspiration
1. Introduction
   a. Common in infants and toddlers because of narrow airway and curiosity
   b. Most commonly involves food, toy, or environmental agent
   c. Dried bean aspiration poses the greatest danger because beans absorb respiratory moisture and form an obstruction; peanuts cause immediate emphysema reaction
   d. Most small objects end up in the right bronchus because it is straighter and wider than the left
2. Assessment
   a. Assess for respiratory distress
   b. Assist with examination of mouth and throat to locate the foreign body
   c. Be aware that the object may be expelled spontaneously
3. Interventions
   a. Perform Heimlich maneuver if the airway is occluded
   b. Assist with measures to open airway, if necessary, such as tracheotomy or intubation
   c. Assist with foreign body removal
   d. Assist with bronchoscopy, if necessary

N. Sudden infant death syndrome (SIDS)
1. Introduction
   a. The sudden unexpected death of a young child in which a postmortem examination fails to demonstrate an adequate cause of death
   b. Syndrome cannot be prevented; is unexpected

     c. Peak age is 3 months; 90% of cases occur before age 6 months

     d. Syndrome unexplained; infant usually dies during sleep without noise or struggle

     e. Autopsy findings indicate pulmonary edema, intrathoracic petechiae, and other minor changes suggesting a chronic hypoxia

2. Assessment

     a. Review family history to see if any siblings were SIDS victims

     b. Review patient's history for low birth weight

3. Interventions

     a. Be aware that since the child is dead, assessment, planning, and implementation of the parents' needs begin as soon as they arrive in the emergency department

     b. Provide family with a room and a health care member; support them and reinforce that this was *not* their fault

     c. Prepare family for how the infant will look and feel

     d. Let parents touch, hold, and rock the infant, if desired; allow them to say good-bye to infant

     e. Prepare parents for autopsy, which is the only way to diagnose SIDS

     f. Contact clergy, significant others, support systems, and local SIDS organization

     g. Provide literature on SIDS and support groups

     h. Suggest psychological support for surviving children

Points to Remember

The respiratory system is immature at birth, even for the normal newborn; the narrow airway predisposes the young child to complications of respiratory illnesses.

The symptoms of and treatments for various conditions resulting in respiratory distress have many similarities.

Asthma is an allergic response resulting in bronchoconstriction; cystic fibrosis is an autosomal recessive disorder resulting in occlusion of the airway by the continuous formation of mucus.

Glossary

Accessory muscles—thoracic and abdominal muscles used during respiratory distress to help expand and contract the chest so the child can inhale and exhale

Air trapping—the inability of the lungs to completely exhale inspired air, leaving air in the lungs

Surfactant—a phospholipid that lines the alveoli, preventing them from collapsing during exhalation

Altered Cardiac Functioning

Learning Objectives

After studying this section, the reader should be able to:

- Differentiate between cyanotic and acyanotic heart defects.

- Assess and plan care for children with cyanotic and acyanotic defects.

- Describe the criteria for determining rheumatic fever.

VIII. Altered Cardiac Functioning

A. Basic concepts: Cardiac pressures

1. After birth, pressure on the left side of the heart is higher than on the right side, with the highest internal pressure in the left ventricle
2. In most cardiac anomalies involving communication between chambers, blood will flow from areas of high pressure to areas of lower pressure; this is called a left-to-right shunt
3. In communicating structures that do not involve chambers, such as patent ductus arteriosus, blood will also flow from high- to low-pressure areas
4. Increased flow to the right side causes hypertrophy of tissue from increased pressure and increased blood flow to the lungs
5. The pressure eventually equalizes between chambers, and the right side will fail in its attempt to compensate

B. Cyanotic heart defects

1. Introduction
   a. The result of any cardiac anomaly in which deoxygenated blood entering the aorta and eventual systemic circulation is mixed with oxygenated blood
   b. The defects can result from any defect causing increased pulmonary vascular resistance resulting in a right-to-left shunt or structural defects allowing the aorta to receive blood from the right side of the heart
   c. Cyanotic heart defects result in left-sided heart failure, a decreased oxygen supply to the body, and the development of collateral circulation
2. Assessment
   a. Observe for cyanosis
   b. Assess for increased pulse and respiratory rate
   c. Note that complete blood count (CBC) will show polycythemia
   d. Review history for irritability and poor feeding
   e. Observe for clubbing of digits
   f. Observe that child may naturally assume a squatting position
   g. Note alterations in blood gas measurements
3. Interventions
   a. Organize and plan care as you would for the anemic child (see Anemia)
   b. Provide oxygen; decrease oxygen demands on child by anticipating needs and preventing distress
   c. Use preemie nipple to decrease energy needed for sucking
   d. Do not interfere when child is squatting; as long as child appears comfortable, no intervention is required other than observation
   e. Provide passive stimulation
   f. Provide good skin care
   g. Prepare child for cardiac catheterization

C. Transposition of the great vessels/arteries (TGA)
   1. Introduction
      a. Cyanotic heart defect
      b. Aorta arises from the right ventricle; pulmonary artery arises from the left ventricle
      c. Deoxygenated blood recirculates from system to right side of the heart and back to the system; oxygenated blood recirculates from the lungs to the left side of the heart and back to the lungs
      d. The child will not survive without communication between these two systems
   2. Assessment
      a. Increasing cyanosis as foramen ovale closes; foramen may remain open longer due to alteration in pressures in the heart
      b. Note other symptoms of a cyanotic heart defect
   3. Interventions
      a. Prepare child for cardiac catheterization
      b. Expect use of prostaglandin E to keep ductus arteriosus open
      c. Prepare child for possible prophylactic surgery to provide communication between chambers
      d. Prepare child for possible corrective surgery (mustard procedure) to redirect blood flow; performed around age 1

D. Tetralogy of Fallot
   1. Introduction
      a. Cyanotic heart defect
      b. Defect consists of pulmonary artery stenosis, ventricular septal defect (VSD), hypertrophy of the right ventricle, and an overriding aorta
      c. Aorta is shifted to the right and receives blood from both the right and left ventricles
      d. Pulmonic stenosis reduces blood flow to lungs; blood with a low oxygen concentration exits into the systemic circulation
      e. Condition stems from increased pressure in the right ventricle; blood shunts right to left, forcing deoxygenated blood to the left side and up the aorta
   2. Assessment
      a. Observe for cyanosis
      b. Note polycythemia
      c. Observe for posturing such as squatting or knee-chest position
      d. Note dyspnea, clubbing of digits, failure to thrive, exercise intolerance, and other symptoms of cyanotic heart disease
      e. Be aware that infants may have episodes of increasing cyanosis, leading to loss of consciousness ("tet spells")
   3. Interventions
      a. Prepare for cardiac catheterization

    b. Prepare for possible palliative treatment to increase blood flow to lungs by bypassing pulmonic stenosis; Blalock-Taussig anastomosis of right pulmonary artery to the right subclavian artery

    c. Be aware that repair of VSD and stenosis may be done in stages

    d. Begin other interventions as for cyanotic heart defects (see Cyanotic heart defects)

E. Hypoplastic left heart syndrome

  1. Introduction

    a. Cyanotic heart defect

    b. The fourth most common cardiac defect

    c. Defect consists of aortic valve atresia, mitral atresia or stenosis, diminutive or absent left ventricle, and severe hypoplasia of the ascending aorta and aortic arch

  2. Interventions

    a. Prepare child for cardiac catheterization

    b. Expect use of prostaglandin E to keep ductus arteriosus patent

    c. Prepare child for surgical intervention (Fontan procedure), which allows use of the right atria as a pumping chamber for pulmonary circulation and the right ventricle as a systemic pumping chamber

    d. Be aware that death will occur in early infancy without surgery

F. Acyanotic heart defects

  1. Introduction

    a. The result of any condition or cardiac anomaly in which blood entering the aorta is completely oxygenated

    b. Acyanotic heart defects include any defect in septa of heart that results in a left-to-right shunt; any increased blood volume on right side of heart that causes right-sided hypertrophy and increased blood flow to lungs; also include any defect between structures that inhibits blood flow to the periphery or results in altered pulmonary resistance

    c. An acyanotic defect can result in cyanosis if the right side of the heart fails and/or not enough oxygenated blood enters circulation

  2. Assessment

    a. Assess for respiratory distress, congested cough, and diaphoresis, which may indicate congestive heart failure (CHF) from increased blood flow to lungs

    b. Note increases in pulse and respiratory rate to compensate for increased blood flow to lungs; assess vital signs

    c. Check for hepatomegaly, since blood can't enter the right side of the heart and backs up in the liver

    d. Review history for frequent respiratory infections from increased pulmonary secretions

    e. Assess for poor growth and development from increased energy expenditure for breathing

    f. Evaluate degree of fatigue

3. Interventions
   a. Expect to administer a digitalis preparation to decrease pulse rate and increase the strength of cardiac contractions; bradycardia is a pulse less than 100 in infants
   b. Monitor fluid status: administer diuretics such as furosemide (Lasix), and observe for potassium loss; enforce fluid restrictions; monitor intake and output, including weighing diapers; obtain daily weight measurements
   c. Reduce oxygen demands by organizing physical care and anticipating child's needs; give high-calorie foods that are easy to ingest and digest
   d. Prevent cold stress by maintaining normal body temperature
   e. Prevent infection
   f. Raise head of bed to ease respiratory status
   g. Prepare child for cardiac catheterization

G. Patent ductus arteriosus (PDA)
1. Introduction
   a. An acyanotic defect resulting from failure of the fetal structure to close; common in premature infants
   b. Blood is shunted to the pulmonary artery (because pressure in the aorta is higher than in the pulmonary artery), which thus increases blood flow to the lungs
2. Assessment
   a. Be aware that the child may be asymptomatic except for a machine-like heart murmur
   b. Assess for signs and symptoms of CHF and left ventricular hypertrophy
3. Interventions
   a. Prepare child for cardiac catheterization
   b. Prepare for possible administration of the prostaglandin inhibitor indomethacin to achieve pharmacologic closure
   c. Prepare for possible surgical correction, which involves ligating the PDA in a closed-heart operation

H. Ventricular septal defect (VSD)
1. Introduction
   a. An acyanotic defect; the most common congenital cardiac anomaly
   b. Defect occurs when a septum fails to complete its formation between the ventricles
   c. Defect results in left-to-right shunt
2. Assessment
   a. Assess for signs and symptoms of CHF with right ventricular hypertrophy
   b. Assess for failure to thrive
   c. Evaluate degree of fatigue
   d. Review history for recurrent respiratory infections

3. Interventions
   a. Prepare child for cardiac catheterization
   b. Prepare for possible pulmonary artery banding to prevent CHF; permanent correction with a patch is performed later, when the heart is larger
   c. Be aware that some children experience spontaneous closure of VSD by age 3

I. Atrial septal defect (ASD)
   1. Introduction
      a. An acyanotic defect
      b. Defect stems from a patent foramen ovale or failure of a septum to completely develop between the atria
      c. Defect results in a left-to-right shunt
   2. Assessment
      a. Assess for signs and symptoms of CHF
      b. Be aware that child may be asymptomatic except for a heart murmur
   3. Interventions
      a. Prepare child for cardiac catheterization
      b. Mild defects may close spontaneously
      b. Prepare child for surgical correction, which involves patching the hole

J. Pulmonic stenosis (PS)
   1. Introduction
      a. An acyanotic defect
      b. Defect involves narrowing or fusing of valves at entrance of pulmonary artery interfering with right ventricular outflow; may result in right ventricular hypertrophy and right heart failure
   2. Assessment
      a. Review history for exertional fatigue
      b. Ask about chest pain with exercise, which occurs in mild to moderate PS
      c. Ask about cyanosis with exercise, which occurs in severe PS
      d. Auscultate for systolic murmur
   3. Interventions
      a. Prepare child for cardiac catheterization
      b. Prepare child for open-heart surgery to separate the pulmonary valve leaflets; will leave the child with a permanent residual murmur

K. Aortic stenosis (AS)
   1. Introduction
      a. An acyanotic defect
      b. Defect involves narrowing or fusion of aortic valves; interferes with left ventricular outflow; may cause left ventricular hypertrophy and left heart failure
      c. AS may progress to include pulmonary congestion

2. Assessment
   a. Ask about syncope and dizziness
   b. Review history for angina
   c. Ask if activities result in an increase in symptoms
   d. Find out what measures brought relief
3. Interventions
   a. Prepare child for cardiac catheterization to assess the degree of AS
   b. Prepare child for surgical palliation with a valvulotomy/commissurotomy; however, this does not prevent stenosis from recurring in adulthood

L. Coarctation of the aorta
1. Introduction
   a. An acyanotic defect
   b. A narrowing of the aortic arch, usually distal to the ductus arteriosus beyond the left subclavian artery
   c. Defect results in decreased blood flow to trunk and lower extremities and increased blood flow to head and arms
   d. Defect predisposes child to cerebrovascular accident (stroke)
2. Assessment
   a. Assess for full bounding pulses in arms, weak or absent pulses in legs; but same pulse rates in both areas
   b. Review history for nosebleeds, headaches, dizziness, leg cramps, and lack of energy
   c. Assess for increased blood pressure in arms, decreased blood pressure in legs
   d. Palpate for warm upper body and cool lower body
   e. Assess for signs and symptoms of CHF from backup pressure to left side of heart
3. Interventions
   a. Prepare child for cardiac catheterization
   b. Expect use of prostaglandin E to keep ductus arteriosus open if infant is dependent on PDA for adequate systemic blood flow
   c. Be aware that if coarctation is proximal to the ductus arteriosus, it is inoperable; surgery for coarctation distal to the ductus arteriosus may involve closed-heart resection of the coarcted portion; this is usually not performed until late preschool age

M. Rheumatic fever (RF)
1. Introduction
   a. An autoimmune immune-complex disorder occurring 1 to 3 weeks after a group A beat-hemolytic streptococci infection, in many cases, after strep throat not treated with penicillin
   b. Antibodies are made against the toxin of the streptococci but attack the heart valves because of similarities in their antigenic markers
   c. Condition results in antigen-antibody complexes that initiate the complement reaction and attack the heart valves

    d. Strep infection *does not* occur in the heart

    e. Disease occurs 7 to 35 days after strep infection; 1% to 5% of patients develop rheumatic fever

  2. Assessment

    a. Use Jones criteria when assessing for RF: major manifestations include carditis, polyarthritis, chorea, subcutaneous nodules, erythema marginatum

    b. Use Jones criteria when assessing for RF: minor manifestations include history of previous RF, fever, arthralgia, increased erythrocyte sedimentation rate, altered electrocardiogram (EKG) with a prolonged PR interval, evidence of a strep infection (elevated antistreptolysin-O [ASO] titer)

  3. Interventions

    a. Administer prophylactic penicillin to prevent additional damage from future attacks; taken until age 20 or for 5 years after attack, whichever is longer

    b. Maintain bed rest until sedimentation rate normalizes

    c. Administer aspirin for discomfort of arthritis

    d. Institute safety measures for chorea: keep a calm environment, reduce stimulation, avoid use of forks or glass, assist in walking

    e. Maintain growth and development with appropriate passive stimulation

    f. Provide emotional support for long-term convalescence

    g. Prevent reinfection

N. Diagnostic and treatment modalities

  1. Cardiac catheterization

    a. Prepare children by using doll play and hospital play; stress the familiar, and make security object available

    b. Describe sensations; do not use the words "injection of dye" but rather "special medicine"

    c. Establish baseline data before the procedure; weigh patient; check color, pulse pressure, and temperature of extremities; check activity level

    d. Keep affected extremity immobile after catheterization to prevent hemorrhage

    e. Monitor after catheterization; check vital signs, color and temperature of extremities; compare all four extremities; compare data to precatheterization baseline data

  2. Cardiac surgery

    a. Prepare child and parents for the sights and sounds of the intensive care unit: chest tubes, breathing exercises, oxygen masks and tents, and other equipment

    b. Perform standard postoperative nursing procedures

Points to Remember

Cyanotic heart defects usually result in cyanosis, polycythemia, and posturing such as squatting.

Acyanotic heart defects usually result in respiratory distress from congestive heart failure.

Rheumatic fever is an acquired but preventable cardiac disease.

Glossary

Acyanotic heart defect—any cardiac anomaly in which blood entering the aorta is completely oxygenated (examples: ASD, VSD)

Chorea—purposeless, rapid, involuntary movements seen as a consequence of rheumatic fever and lasting for months

Cyanotic heart defect—any cardiac anomaly in which deoxygenated blood entering the aorta and systemic circulation is mixed with oxygenated blood (examples: tetralogy of Fallot, TGA)

Left-to-right shunt—pressure on the left side of the heart pushing blood through a septal defect to the right side, thus increasing blood flow to the lungs

Altered Gastrointestinal Functioning

Learning Objectives

After studying this section, the reader should be able to:

• Describe acquired and congenital gastrointestinal problems that alter nutrition and hydration.

• Assess and plan care for the child with vomiting and/or diarrhea.

• Plan feeding interventions for the child with congenital anomalies that interfere with ingesting nutrients.

• Distinguish congenital anomalies from acquired inflammatory processes of the gastrointestinal tract.

IX. Altered Gastrointestinal Functioning

A. Basic concepts

1. Many gastrointestinal abnormalities originate during fetal life
2. The abnormalities may or may not be detected early in infancy
3. Signs and symptoms will depend on which part of the gastrointestinal tract is affected

B. Vomiting

1. Introduction
    a. This forceful emptying of the stomach contents through the mouth results from such conditions as spasm of the duodenum; reverse peristalsis resulting from blockage of the pylorus; reflux from an incompetent lax esophageal sphincter, overdistention of the stomach resulting from increased intake or gastroenteritis, or nongastrointestinal disorders, such as increased intracranial pressure
    b. The medulla controls vomiting
    c. Spitting up or wet burps involve either dribbling of undigested liquids from the mouth and esophagus or expulsion with the force of a burp
2. Assessment
    a. Differentiate vomiting from a wet burp
    b. Note history of vomiting and frequency of vomiting episodes
    c. Assess for other symptoms that accompany it, such as fever, nausea, headache, diarrhea
    d. Determine if it is projectile
    e. Determine if it is related to intake or other activities
    f. Describe vomitus: blood, bile, undigested or digested food, amount, force
    g. Check for bowel sounds
    h. Assess hydration status; assess electrolyte balance
    i. Assess for metabolic alkalosis from loss of stomach acids
    j. Assess nutritional status
    k. Evaluate feeding methods (amount of burping, air in nipple)
3. Interventions
    a. Prevent aspiration by positioning child on side; maintain patent airway; nasotracheal or bulb suctioning may be necessary
    b. Withhold food and fluids to rest stomach
    c. If cause is not obstructive, replace fluids after a period of withholding food and fluids; use I.V. fluids or start with small amounts of clear liquid orally, then progress to tea and ginger ale
    d. Administer antiemetic medications; use the rectal or intramuscular route
    e. Test emesis for blood
    f. Measure amount of emesis after each vomiting episode
    g. Raise head of bed when feeding
    h. Provide skin and mouth care
    i. Monitor hydration status, such as daily weight and intake and output
    j. Monitor bowel status

C. Gastroesophageal reflux (GER)/chalasia
1. Introduction
   a. Return of gastric contents into the esophagus from incompetent or poorly developed esophageal sphincter
   b. Occurs most commonly during infancy
   c. Occurs almost immediately after eating
2. Assessment
   a. Assess relationship of vomiting to feedings, positioning, and activity level immediately after feeding
   b. Assess for failure to thrive
   c. Assess for aspiration of feedings, and note any relationship between apnea and GER
   d. Measure pH of gastric contents
3. Interventions
   a. Administer thickened formula, since thinner formula is refluxed easier
   b. Feed in upright position and keep upright for 1 hour after feedings
   c. Give small, frequent feedings
   d. Be aware that a surgical procedure may be necessary: Nissen fundoplication

D. Diarrhea/gastroenteritis
1. Introduction
   a. Increased frequency and amount and decreased consistency of stool
   b. Increased water in bowel from osmotic pull, electrolyte imbalance, or an increase in peristalsis, which prevents water from being absorbed
   c. May be due to virus or bacteria in the GI tract
   d. Can result in metabolic acidosis and dehydration
   e. Other causes: malabsorption, anatomic changes, GI allergies, toxins, and inflammation of the bowel
2. Assessment
   a. Note amount, frequency, duration, consistency, appearance, odor of stool; weigh diapers and note amount of water loss
   b. Test stools for blood and other reducing substances, such as sugars, and for pH
   c. Ask whether abdominal pain or cramping is associated with stooling
   d. Assess relationship between stooling and the time of eating or quality of intake
   e. Observe skin integrity around the anus
   f. Expect to rule out other conditions that may cause diarrhea
   g. Assess hydration status; be alert for alteration in CNS functioning
   h. Check bowel sounds; get stool cultures, if ordered
3. Interventions
   a. Withhold food and fluids to rest bowel
   b. Administer kaolin and pectin (Kaopectate) to make stools firmer for the older child; paregoric (an opiate) will decrease bowel motility

    c. Correct dehydration; replace potassium
    d. Begin fluid intake with an electrolyte-balanced solution such as Pedialyte
    e. Avoid solutions that are high in sodium (broth, milk) because of their osmotic pull
    f. Progress to BRAT diet (bread, rice cereal, applesauce, weak tea)
    g. Practice enteric precautions, good handwashing
    h. Measure urine and stool output; use pediatric plastic urine collector around the urethra to catch urine, if necessary
    i. Use prophylactic or therapeutic skin care around anus with protective ointments
    j. Do not take temperature rectally; use axillary method

E. Constipation
  1. Introduction
    a. Decreased amount and increased consistency of stools, compared to the child's normal pattern
    b. Children do not need to have a bowel movement every day
    c. Condition may be due to a diet low in liquids and high in fat and protein
    d. Straining is not necessarily synonymous with constipation
  2. Assessment
    a. Note hard, dry, infrequent stool
    b. Test stool for blood; possible hematest-positive stool from trauma to rectal tissue from passing hard mass; assess skin integrity around anus
    c. Ask about abdominal pain while stooling and/or intermittent pain throughout the day
    d. Assess diet for liquids, fiber, carbohydrates, constipating foods
    e. Test stools for reducing substances
    f. Measure abdominal girth
    g. Note whether child is reluctant to use toilet in school or is consciously retaining stool
  3. Interventions
    a. Lubricate around anus to make passage easier during passage of hard stool
    b. Remove stool digitally if necessary
    c. Administer stool softeners: suppositories, mineral oil, docusate sodium (Colace)
    d. Add Karo syrup to formula
    e. Add fiber or prune juice to diet
    f. Administer enemas; use isotonic solutions only

F. Cleft lip and palate
  1. Introduction
    a. Failure of bone and tissue of upper jaw and palate to fuse at the midline; incomplete fusion
    b. Can be inherited or congenital; cleft may be partial or complete; a unilateral or bilateral cleft of the lip, palate, or both may occur

    c. Requires a long-term team approach to address speech defects, dental and orthodontic problems, nasal defects, and possible alterations in hearing

    d. Results in facial disfigurement; parental shock, guilt, and grief upon seeing infant may result; condition may block parental bonding with child

    e. May have nasal distortion

    f. Increased open space in mouth causes some formula to exit through nose with wet burps; infant is more prone to aspiration

    g. Increase in open space in oropharynx decreases natural defenses against bacterial invasion, leading to increased risk of upper respiratory infection or otitis media

2. Assessment

    a. Assess quality of child's sucking by putting examiner's finger in infant's mouth; determine if infant can form an airtight seal around finger or nipple

    b. Assess ability to swallow

    c. Assess for abdominal distention from swallowed air

    d. Be alert for respiratory distress when feeding

3. Interventions for cleft lip (preoperative)

    a. Feed neonate slowly and in an upright position to decrease risk of aspiration

    b. Burp often during feeding to eliminate air swallowed and decrease risk of emesis

    c. Use long soft lamb's nipple, cleft palate nipple with a flap across palate, medicine dropper, syringe with rubber tubing attached to end, and/or manual compression to unite the edges of the cleft lip; all are methods to encourage sucking, promote oral muscle development, and enhance the nutritional status

    d. Use gavage feedings if oral feedings are unsuccessful

    e. Administer a small amount of water after feedings to prevent formula from accumulating and becoming a medium for bacterial growth

    f. Administer feedings in small, frequent portions

    g. Hold while feeding, and promote sucking between meals

    h. Provide psychological support to parents; reinforce success of surgery

    i. Tell parents that cleft lips are usually corrected when the infant is 10 weeks old and weighs 10 pounds (4.5 kg); child must be free of respiratory infections at time of surgery

4. Interventions for cleft lip repair (cheiloplasty) (postoperative)

    a. Be aware that procedure unites the lip and gum edges in anticipation of teeth eruption, provides a route for adequate nutrition and sucking, and improves the child's appearance, which promotes parental-child bonding

    b. Maintain a patent airway; do not position prone; edema and/or narrowing of a previously large airway may make the child appear to be in distress

    c. Observe for cyanosis as child begins to breathe through nose

    d. Maintain intact suture line; keep child's hands away from mouth by using restraints or pinning sleeves to shirt

   e. Prevent tension on suture line by anticipating infant's needs and preventing crying
   f. Give extra TLC since child cannot meet his emotional needs by sucking
   g. When feeding resumes, use syringe with tubing to administer foods at side of mouth; this will prevent trauma to the suture line
   h. After feedings, place child on right side to prevent aspiration
   i. Clean suture line after each feeding by dabbing with half-strength peroxide or saline solution to prevent crusts and scarring
   j. Monitor and treat for pain
5. Interventions for cleft palate (preoperative)
   a. Be aware that child must be weaned from bottle or breast before cleft palate surgery; must be able to drink from a cup
   b. Feed child with a cleft palate nipple or a teflon implant to enhance nutritional intake
   c. Tell the parents that surgery will be scheduled at about age 18 months to allow for growth of the palate and before child develops speech patterns; child must be free from ear and respiratory infections
   d. Teach parents that child is susceptible to pathogens and otitis media from altered position of eustachian tubes
6. Interventions for cleft palate repair (staphylorrhaphy) (postoperative)
   a. Maintain patent airway; position child on abdomen or side
   b. Anticipate edema and a decrease in the size of the airway due to closure of the palate; this may make child appear dyspneic
   c. Prevent trauma to suture line by keeping hard or pointed objects away from mouth, for example, utensils, straws, popsicle sticks
   d. Use cup to feed
   e. Use elbow restraints to keep hands from mouth
   f. Provide soft toys
   g. Start on clear liquids and progress to soft diet; rinse suture line with a sip of water after each feeding
   h. Distract child or hold him to try to keep tongue away from roof of mouth

G. Esophageal atresia and tracheoesophageal fistula
1. Introduction
   a. Atresia means termination of a passageway; it usually refers to a pathologic closure or absence of a normal anatomic opening
   b. A fistula is a tubelike connection between two structures
   c. These conditions occur in many combinations and are common in premature infants; may be associated with other defects
   d. Esophageal atresia (EA) occurs when the proximal end of esophagus ends in a blind pouch; food cannot enter stomach via esophagus
   e. Tracheoesophageal fistula (TEF) occurs when a connection exists between the esophagus and the trachea
   f. TEF may result in reflux of gastric juice after feeding that can allow acidic stomach contents to cross the fistula, irritating the trachea

g. EA with TEF occurs when the distal end of the esophagus ends in a blind pouch; proximal end of the esophagus is linked to the trachea via a fistula

2. Assessment of EA
   a. Assess for excessive salivation and drooling from inability to pass food through esophagus
   b. Note that a nasogastric tube cannot be passed
   c. Observe for regurgitation of undigested formula immediately after feeding; respiratory distress and cyanosis may occur if secretions are aspirated

3. Assessment of TEF
   a. Assess for choking and intermittent cyanosis during feeding from food that goes through the fistula into the trachea
   b. Observe for abdominal distention from air that goes through the fistula into the stomach

4. Assessment of EA with TEF
   a. Note that all signs and symptoms of esophageal atresia are also seen with this anomaly
   b. Observe for signs of severe respiratory distress—coughing, choking, and cyanosis—since the infant is in danger of drowning immediately after swallowing any material

5. Interventions for anomalies of the esophagus
   a. Do not feed orally if any of these signs occur
   b. Feed all newborns first with a few sips of sterile water to prevent aspiration of formula into the lungs
   c. Maintain a patent airway; have suction equipment available
   d. When feeding child, anticipate abdominal distention from air and crying; burp frequently; keep upright to reduce the chance of reflux of stomach contents and aspiration pneumonia
   e. Teach parents alternative feeding methods, and explain the surgery to ligate the TEF and/or to reanastomose the esophageal ends

H. Pyloric stenosis

1. Introduction
   a. Increasing hyperplasia and hypertrophy of the circular muscle at the pylorus, which narrows the pyloric canal
   b. Defect is commonly seen in children between age 1 and 6 months
   c. Emesis may be hematest-positive but will *not* contain bile; it will increase in amount and force as the obstruction increases and become projectile

2. Assessment
   a. Be aware that symptoms seldom appear during the first few weeks of life
   b. Palpate for an olive-size bulge below the right costal margin
   c. Observe for emesis during or shortly after feedings (preceded by reverse peristaltic waves; it will not be preceded by nausea)

    d. Note that child will resume eating after vomiting

    e. Evaluate for poor weight gain and symptoms of malnutrition despite child's apparent hunger

    f. Assess for metabolic alkalosis and dehydration from frequent emesis

    g. Observe for projectile vomiting

  3. Interventions

    a. Provide small, frequent, thickened feedings with head of bed elevated; burp frequently

    b. Position to prevent aspiration of vomitus; placing child on right side is preferred

    c. Correct electrolyte imbalance

    d. Prepare for surgery (pyloromyotomy)

I. Intussusception

  1. Introduction

    a. Telescoping or invagination of bowel segment into itself

    b. May be from polyps, hyperactive peristalsis, or abnormal lining of the bowel

    c. Causes inflammation and swelling of affected portion of bowel; edema eventually causes obstruction and necrosis from occlusion of blood supply to bowel

    d. Most common at about age 6 months

    e. If untreated, peritonitis may develop

    f. Can be acute or chronic; begins as episodic and progresses to total obstruction

  2. Assessment of acute attack

    a. Note sudden attack of acute abdominal pain; shrieking screams; knees drawn to chest

    b. Observe for increase in bile-stained vomitus

    c. Note passage of red currant jelly–like stool

    d. Assess for distended and tender abdomen

    e. Note pallor and agitation

  3. Interventions

    a. Prepare for barium enema to confirm condition and reduce the invagination by hydrostatic pressure

    b. Be aware that, if reduction by barium fails, surgery may be required to resect the gangrenous portion and make a temporary colostomy

J. Congenital aganglionic megacolon (Hirschsprung's disease)

  1. Introduction

    a. Absence of parasympathetic ganglionic cells in a segment of colon, causing a lack or alteration in peristalsis in the affected part

    b. As stool enters the affected part, it remains there until additional stool pushes it through; affected part of colon dilates; may result in a mechanical obstruction

    c. Usually occurs at distal end of large intestine

2. Assessment
   a. Observe newborn for failure to pass meconium and stool
   b. Observe for liquid or ribbonlike stools, since only fluid can pass the obstruction caused by stool
   c. Assess for distended abdomen from stool impaction
   d. Assess for nausea, bile-stained vomitus, anorexia, lethargy, weight loss, failure to thrive
   e. Prepare for rectal biopsy to confirm the condition
   f. Be alert for signs and symptoms of enterocolitis, volvulus, and shock, which can occur from the disease
3. Interventions
   a. Perform a digital exam to expand the anus enough to release impacted stool and provide temporary relief if the megacolon is near the rectum
   b. Do not treat liquid stool as diarrhea; it is the result of impaction
   c. Administer isotonic enemas (saline solution or mineral oil) to evacuate the bowel
   d. Be aware that total parenteral nutrition may be used in place of oral feedings in order to rest the bowel
   e. Use low-residue diets and stool softeners to lessen stool bulk and thus decrease the irritation to the colon
   f. Be aware that surgery may be required to remove the aganglionic section and make a temporary colostomy

K. Imperforate anus
1. Introduction
   a. Atresia of anal opening; may have no anal opening onto skin wall; rectum may end in blind pouch
   b. A fistula to vagina in females or to urethra in males may also be present
2. Assessment
   a. Observe to see from which orifice stool is excreted
   b. Assess for signs and symptoms of impaction from inability to pass stool
   c. Insertion of a rectal thermometer may not be possible
3. Interventions
   a. Do not take temperature rectally; use axillary method
   b. After surgical reconstruction of the anus and formation of a temporary colostomy, keep infant prone with hips elevated

L. Appendicitis
1. Introduction
   a. Inflammation and obstruction of blind sac at end of cecum, resulting in ischemia, gangrene, perforation, and peritonitis
   b. Suggested causes include infections, dietary intake, constipation, and parasites
   c. Common in school-age children

2. Assessment
    a. Remember that symptoms are variable, making a quick and accurate diagnosis difficult
    b. Assess for abdominal pain and tenderness that begins as diffuse, then localizes in the lower right quadrant at McBurney's point
    c. Note fever, increased white blood cell count, behavioral changes
    d. Note rebound tenderness, especially in the lower right quadrant
    e. Assess for decreased bowel sounds, nausea, vomiting, anorexia
    f. Assess for abdominal rigidity and guarding
    g. Note symptoms of peritonitis if rupture occurs
3. Interventions
    a. Position preoperatively in a semi-Fowler or right side-lying position
    b. Be aware that, postoperatively, child has a Penrose drain and a nasogastric (NG) tube attached to low intermittent suction; periodically irrigate tube
    c. Resume oral nutrition when bowel sounds reappear
    d. Administer antibiotics

M. Inflammatory bowel disease
1. Introduction
    a. Includes Crohn's disease (regional enteritis) and ulcerative colitis
    b. Diagnosed by barium enema, biopsy of the GI mucosa, and stool studies
    c. Involves edema and inflammation of bowel resulting in ulceration, bleeding, diarrhea, and abdominal distention
    d. Involves chronic exacerbations that may delay growth and development, including sexual development
    e. Occurs more commonly in adolescents
    f. Exacerbated by emotional factors, but cause is unknown
2. Assessment
    a. Assess for weight loss, anorexia, nausea, and vomiting
    b. Test stool for blood
    c. Observe for diarrhea
    d. Test for anemia from bleeding
3. Interventions
    a. Administer analgesics and antispasmodics to decrease abdominal pain
    b. Administer corticosteroids to decrease bowel inflammation
    c. Promote stress reduction through relaxation, distraction, enhanced self-image and self-esteem
    d. Withhold food and fluids using parenteral nutrition in place of feeding to rest the bowel, or provide high-protein, high-calorie, low-residue, and low-fat diet
    e. Be aware that when conditions are not amenable to medical treatment, a temporary colostomy or ileostomy may be performed

    4. Differences between ulcerative colitis (UC) and Crohn's disease
      a. UC involves symmetrical and contiguous GI ulcers; Crohn's disease involves asymmetrical and patchy lesions
      b. UC causes more blood loss than Crohn's disease
      c. UC attacks the mucosa of the bowel; Crohn's disease affects all layers of the bowel wall
      d. Crohn's disease involves enlarged regional lymph nodes
      e. UC usually involves the large intestine; Crohn's disease can occur at any point along the GI tract

N. Celiac disease
    1. Introduction
      a. Absence of enzyme in intestinal mucosal cells causes atrophy of villi of proximal small intestine and decreases the absorptive capacity of the intestines
      b. An effect of a gluten intolerance; inability to absorb rye, oat, wheat, and barley glutens
      c. Related to IgA deficiency and early introduction of protein solids; usually occurs 2 to 4 months after solid foods are introduced
    2. Assessment
      a. Assess for steatorrhea and chronic diarrhea from malabsorption of fats
      b. Assess for generalized malnutrition and failure to thrive from malabsorption of protein and carbohydrates
      c. Evaluate for osteoporosis and coagulation difficulty from malabsorption of fat-soluble vitamins
      d. Assess for abdominal pain from calcium depletion
      e. Observe for irritability from anemia
      f. Prepare for intestinal biopsy to diagnose the condition
    3. Interventions
      a. Eliminate gluten from the diet
      b. Give corn and rice products, soy and potato flour, Probana formula, and all fresh fruits
      c. Replace vitamins and calories; give small, frequent meals
      d. Prevent the disease by delaying introduction of solid foods until after age 6 months

O. Biliary atresia
    1. Introduction
      a. Obliteration, atresia, or absence of extrahepatic biliary structures
      b. Defect occurs shortly before birth
      c. Cause undetermined
      d. Liver failure and death can result
    2. Assessment
      a. Observe for jaundice early in infancy
      b. Observe for dark urine and pale stools from absence of bile

    c. Assess for hepatomegaly, ascites, splenomegaly
    d. Expect irritability
    e. Assess for failure to thrive or poor weight gain from decreased absorption of fat-soluble vitamins
    f. Note that lab tests show increased conjugated bilirubin, cholesterol, and alkaline phosphatase and prolonged prothrombin time
    g. Prepare for liver biopsy to diagnose the condition

3. Interventions
    a. Give fat-soluble vitamins in water-miscible form
    b. Be aware that, if no treatable condition is identified, surgery (Kasai procedure) can be done to form a substitute duct, but this is not a permanent correction
    c. Be aware that a liver transplant may be done for uncorrectable atresia

P. Hernias

1. Introduction
    a. Muscle weakness, causing protrusion of an organ through the abnormal musculature
    b. Umbilical hernia: weakness in the umbilical area, where umbilical blood vessels traveled; failure of umbilical muscles to close at birth, resulting in protrusion of omentum and intestine through the naval
    c. Inguinal canal hernias: weakness where testes descended from abdomen to scrotum and where the proximal portion of the inguinal canal failed to atrophy and protrudes through the inguinal canal

2. Assessment
    a. Assess for increase in size of lump as patient strains, coughs, or cries
    b. Note that condition is usually present without pain

3. Interventions
    a. Observe for symptoms of incarceration
    b. Tell parents that home measures such as belly bands and abdominal binders are not effective
    c. Remember that the abdominal muscles often strengthen as the child grows and the hernia may resolve without treatment
    d. Be aware that, if hernia does not resolve, surgical intervention may be required; this is usually done in a short-stay unit

Q. Parasitic worms (helminths)

1. Introduction
    a. Worms are obtained by ingesting dirt or raw vegetables containing helminth eggs or acquired through the skin
    b. Eggs hatch and travel by GI tract or blood to gut, where they attach and thrive
    c. They are often a result of unsanitary disposal of stool and absence of handwashing

      d. Symptoms are dependent on worm type and load as well as on degree of intestinal damage and irritation

2. Assessment
   a. Assess for bloody diarrhea leading to anemia; stool is hematest-positive
   b. Assess for failure to thrive related to malabsorption
   c. Assess for abdominal distention, anorexia, nausea and vomiting
   d. Expect possible intense anal pruritus and scratching if infestation with pinworms

3. Interventions
   a. Teach sanitary disposal of stool
   b. Teach handwashing before meals and after toileting
   c. Teach washing of fruits and vegetables before eating
   d. Have children wear shoes in infested areas
   e. Administer appropriate medication depending on type of infestation

4. Pinworm
   a. Most common worm infestation
   b. 5 to 10 mm long
   c. Worms live in cecum and crawl to anus at night to deposit eggs in perianal area
   d. The cycle repeats itself when child scratches anus and puts hand to mouth
   e. Condition can be dignosed by scotch tape test, where tape is put across rectum at night; worms lay eggs on tape; tape can be removed in the morning and used as a microscope slide to diagnose
   f. Oral medication for pinworms will color stool red (not related to bleeding)

Points to Remember

For any gastrointestinal condition that results in emesis, maintaining a patent airway takes priority.

Cleft lip and palate and related esophageal anomalies require adjustments in feeding methods.

Gastrointestinal obstruction can stem from stenosis of the GI tract, altered peristalsis, inflammation, constipation, telescoping of the bowel, or abnormalities in the colon.

Inflammatory gastrointestinal conditions are acquired and irritate the bowel wall.

Glossary

Atresia—termination or absence of a normal anatomic passageway

Cleft—the partial or complete failure of fusion of body structures, such as the lip and palate

Fistula—a tubelike connection between two structures

Inflammatory bowel disease—a generalized classification for conditions that include Crohn's disease and ulcerative colitis and result in ulceration of the bowel

Altered Genitourinary Functioning

Learning Objectives

After studying this section, the reader should be able to:

• Describe how the fluid and electrolyte status of children differs from adults.

• Assess and plan care for the dehydrated child.

• Assess and plan care for a child with infected or inflamed renal and urinary systems.

• Describe congenital anomalies of the genitourinary tract.

X. Altered Genitourinary Functioning

A. Fluid and electrolyte balance in the child

1. Proportion of total body water to body weight
   a. Water is the body's primary fluid; the amount of body water varies with age, sex, and the percentage of body fat
   b. The proportion of body water to body weight decreases with increasing age from development of increased body fat (after puberty, females have more fat than males) and the growth of solid body structures
   c. Adult percentage of body water for men (63%) is attained by age 1 to 3; a premature infant's weight is 90% water, whereas a full-term infant's weight is 75% to 80% water (a woman's body is 52% water)
   d. The distribution of body water does not reach that of the adult until late school-age; infants have much more total body water in the extracellular fluid (42% to 45%) than adults (20%); therefore, they cannot conserve water as well and have less fluid reserve
   e. Because of the increased percentage of water in their extracellular fluid, children's water turnover rate is 2 to 3 times higher than adults' and, therefore, children are more susceptible to dehydration; 50% of the infant's extracellular fluid is exchanged every day, compared to only 20% for the adult

2. Metabolism
   a. Because a child's growth process depends on, and results in, an increased metabolic rate (2 to 3 times that of adults), a child also produces more metabolic waste
   b. A child's pulse, respiratory, and peristaltic rates are higher than an adult's, resulting in a greater proportion of insensible water loss
   c. Young children need more water per kg/body weight than do adults, to replace the insensible water loss resulting from their increased metabolism and the resulting increased amount of metabolic waste

3. Body-surface area
   a. Newborns have a greater ratio of body-surface area to body weight than adults
   b. Shivering and sweating mechanisms are effective after infancy as partial mechanisms to control body temperature
   c. Increased body-surface area results in greater fluid loss through the skin than adults

4. Renal function
   a. Children attain the adult number of nephrons by age 1, although these structures continue to mature throughout early childhood
   b. The infant's renal function can maintain a healthy fluid and electrolyte status; however, it doesn't compensate as efficiently during stress as the adult's
   c. The infant has a low glomerular filtration rate; however, the rate approaches the adult level by age 2

    d. Infants don't concentrate urine at an adult level until after age 2; average specific gravity for infants is less than 1.010 (for an adult, it is 1.010 to 1.030)

    e. The number of daily voidings decreases because of increased concentration of urine, even though the total amount of urine produced daily may not vary significantly

    f. The infant usually voids 5 to 10 ml/hour; a 10-year-old, 10 to 25 ml/hour (an adult voids 35 ml/hour); a 4-year-old's bladder holds 250 ml, allowing him to stay dry through the night

    g. Inefficient reabsorption of sodium can result in hyponatremia

    h. A child has a short urethra, which can easily transmit organisms into the bladder; the female urethra is closer to the rectum than the male's, posing a greater risk of contamination by inappropriate wiping after a bowel movement

5. Urinary function studies

    a. Urine should be checked for blood, protein, glucose, ketones, and pH via a dipstick test; specific gravity should also be checked (urine can be collected from the cotton matting in the diaper)

    b. The clean-catch method should be used to collect urine from an infant; after proper cleaning of skin and genitals, a pediatric urine collector should be applied to dry skin (powders or creams should not be used); if the child does not void within 45 minutes, the bag should be removed and the process repeated

    c. An I.V. pyelogram is done to check renal pelvic structures. (The dye injected before the X-rays are taken should be referred to as a "special medicine")

    d. A voiding cystourethrogram is done to view the bladder and related structures during voiding via instillation of contrast material in the bladder through a catheter; young children cannot retain the fluid, and older children may be frightened and embarrassed as they are ordered to urinate on the X-ray table

    e. Blood urea nitrogen (BUN) level, creatinine level, and glomerular filtration rate are also evaluated

B. The dehydrated child

1. Introduction

    a. Dehydration can occur from decreased intake of fluid or loss of water and electrolytes via vomiting, diarrhea, or diaphoresis; water output exceeds input

    b. Dehydration refers to the percentage of body weight lost as water; it can be severe enough to result in volume depletion, circulatory collapse, and shock

    c. 15% isotonic dehydration in an infant is considered severe; 9% loss in an older child is considered severe

    d. *Isotonic dehydration:* a deficiency of water and electrolytes in approximately equal proportions

    e. *Hypotonic dehydration:* a loss of more electrolytes than water, causing extracellular-to-intracellular movement of water and resulting in shock

    f. *Hypertonic dehydration:* a loss of more water than electrolytes (water-loss dehydration) causing intracellular-to-extracellular movement of fluid and resulting in neurologic changes

2. Assessment

    a. Assess quality and quantity of fluid intake and output; intake may be greater than output but insufficient to meet the body's needs; water may be lost in stool or vomiting

    b. Note decreased urine output and concentrated urine

    c. Note sudden weight loss

    d. Assess for dry skin with poor tissue turgor; sunken fontanel in infant

    e. Assess for decrease in tears and saliva; dry mucous membranes; sunken and soft eyeballs; thirst

    f. Note pale skin with poor perfusion, cool extremities, decreased body temperature, tachycardia, hypotension

    g. Note lethargy and irritability; high-pitched, weak cry

3. Interventions

    a. Record hourly all stools, vomitus, and urine; note amount, color, consistency, concentration, time, relation to meals or stress, and results of specific gravity and other values from urine dipstick tests

    b. Withhold food and fluids and use I.V. replacement of fluids; provide sucking stimulation to young infants

    c. Provide mouth care with lemon and glycerine swabs

    d. Provide skin care; turn every 2 hours and keep extremities warm

    e. Measure intake and output carefully; weigh diapers, record fluids used to take medications; indicate fluid lost by diaphoresis, suctioning, or other tubes

    f. Weigh daily with same scale at same time each day, with child naked or wearing same amount of clothing

    g. Provide rest

    h. Monitor for and prevent shock

    i. When restarting fluids for an infant, give Pedialyte

    j. When restarting fluids for older children, start with flat soda or sweet, weak tea

    k. Note that any increase in the ambient heat or water loss requires greater fluid intake to meet hydration needs

C. Urinary tract infection (UTI)

1. Introduction

    a. Microbial invasion of the urinary tract

     b. UTI is more common in females because of placement and size of
        urethra
     c. UTI may also be caused by reflux, irritation by bubble baths, poor
        hygiene, or incomplete emptying of the bladder
2. Assessment
     a. Assess quantity, quality, and frequency of voiding
     b. Note that clean-catch urine culture will demonstrate large amounts of
        bacteria
     c. Assess for increased pH of urine, hematuria
     d. Ask about frequent urge to void with pain or burning on urination
     e. Note low-grade fever, lethargy, poor feeding
     f. Ask about abdominal pain
     g. Assess for enuresis
     h. Assess toileting habits (Does child wipe front to back? Does he wash his
        hands properly?)
     i. Assess bathing habits (Does child take tub baths, bubble baths?)
     j. Assess number of urinary infections per year; may be recurrent
3. Interventions
     a. Administer antibiotics such as sulfisoxazole (Gantrisin) and ampicillin to
        prevent glomerulonephritis
     b. Force fluids to flush infection from urinary tract
     c. Administer cranberry juice to increase acidity of urine
     d. Teach good toileting hygiene; encourage use of toilet every 2 hours
     e. Discourage tub baths and bubble baths

D. Enuresis
1. Introduction
     a. Repeated involuntary urination after age 5, usually while asleep
     b. Incontinence may occur at night, day, or both; can be primary, where the
        child has never completely been controlled, or secondary, which occurs
        after a period of bladder control
     c. Suggested causes include stress, incomplete muscle maturation, altered
        sleep patterns, or irritable bladder that cannot handle large amounts of
        urine
2. Assessment
     a. Review history for age of toilet training; onset of enuresis; frequency of
        occurrences
     b. Ask about history of previous urinary tract infections; burning on
        urination; sense of urgency
     c. Expect urinalysis, urine culture and sensitivity, and blood studies
        including BUN and creatinine to evaluate renal function
3. Interventions
     a. Be aware that treatment varies with cause
     b. Remind child to use toilet every 2 hours
     c. Decrease fluids after 5 p.m. except to satisfy thirst

    d. Administer imipramine (Tofranil) to inhibit urination

    e. Teach bladder-stretching exercises during the day by having child drink large amounts of fluids; try to keep bladder enlarged for a while before emptying

    f. Provide emotional support to child and parents; do not embarrass or punish

    g. Do not refer to enuresis as an accident, since accidents can be prevented

E. Nephrotic syndrome/nephrosis

  1. Introduction

    a. An autoimmune process that occurs 1 week after an immune assault

    b. Disease increases permeability of the glomerulus to protein, especially albumin

    c. Disease is commonly seen in toddlers

  2. Assessment

    a. Note proteinuria and hypoproteinemia

    b. Assess for signs and symptoms of hypovolemia

    c. Note that morning urine will usually have a high protein level; urine is dark, foamy, and frothy and has a high specific gravity; urine production decreases

    d. Note that only microscopic hematuria will be manifested; no frank bleeding

    e. Assess for dependent body edema with weight gain; periorbital edema in the morning; abdominal ascites and increased abdominal girth; scrotal edema; ankle edema by midday; diarrhea, anorexia, and malnutrition from edema of intestinal mucosa

    f. Check electrolyte levels, since potassium is lost in urine with diuresis

    g. Observe for stretched, shiny skin with a waxy pallor

    h. Be aware of increased susceptibility to infection from increased interstitial fluid

    i. Note fatigue and/or lethargy

    j. Prepare for renal biopsy to diagnose the disease

  3. Interventions

    a. Provide skin care to edematous skin; do not use adhesive strip bandages, tape, or I.M. injections

    b. Provide warm soaks to decrease periorbital edema; elevate head of bed

    c. Turn frequently; provide scrotal support and place padding between body parts to prevent irritation

    d. Test first void of day for protein

    e. Feed small, frequent meals; measure intake and output and daily weight

    f. Administer steroids to suppress the autoimmune response and to stimulate vascular reabsorption of edema

    g. Prevent contact with persons who have an infection

    h. Anticipate diuresis in 1 to 3 weeks; maintain bed rest during rapid diuresis; monitor hydration status and vital signs

F.   Acute glomerulonephritis (AGN)
1.   Introduction
    a.   An autoimmune immune-complex disorder occurring 1 to 2 weeks after a Group A beta-hemolytic streptococci infection
    b.   Antibodies are made against the toxin of the streptococci but attack the glomerulus because of similarities in their antigenic markers
    c.   Condition results in antigen-antibody complexes that initiate the complement reaction and cause renal damage in the glomeruli
    d.   Streptococcus is not present in the kidney at any time
    e.   Common in children ages 4 to 7
2.   Assessment
    a.   Assess for signs and symptoms of altered kidney function from edema and renal damage
    b.   Observe and test urine for hematuria; cola-colored (smoky) urine
    c.   Note decreased urine output
    d.   Note that blood tests show increased sedimentation rate, indicating an inflammatory process; increased ASO titer, indicating a recent streptococcus infection
    e.   Assess for and monitor increased blood pressure
    f.   Note appearance of either periorbital or dependent edema or both
    g.   Irritability, lethargy, and anemic appearance
3.   Interventions
    a.   Implement the same measures as for nephrosis
    b.   Expect possible penicillin therapy and teach parents about possible long-term penicillin therapy to prevent further renal damage in a subsequent streptococcal infection
    c.   Institute moderate sodium restriction for children with hypertension or edema
    d.   Administer medications to control hypertension

G. Hypospadias and epispadias
1.   Introduction
    a.   Hypospadias is a congenital anomaly of the penis; the urethral opening may be anywhere along the ventral side of the penis
    b.   In epispadias, the urethral opening may appear anywhere along the dorsal side of the penis; an uncommon condition associated with exstrophy of the bladder
    c.   Both conditions shorten the distance to the bladder, offering easier access to bacteria
2.   Assessment
    a.   Observe angle of urination
    b.   Observe site of exit
3.   Interventions
    a.   Keep area clean to exclude bacteria
    b.   Do not circumcise an infant with suspected hypospadias; the foreskin may be needed later in the surgical repair

    c. Be aware that surgery involving implants or reconstruction may be needed to reduce the chance of urinary tract infections and infertility

H. Undescended testes (cryptorchidism)

1. Introduction
   a. Testes descend from abdomen into scrotum during last 2 months of gestation
   b. If testes are not descended at birth, they may descend on their own in a few weeks
   c. If testes remain in abdominal cavity after age 5, the seminiferous tubules may degenerate due to the increased body temperature in the abdomen, resulting in sterility
2. Assessment
   a. Palpate scrotum; undescended testes are usually unilateral
   b. Note that other findings are normal on palpation
3. Interventions
   a. Expect diagnostic tests to check kidney function since kidneys and testes arise from the same germ tissue
   b. Be aware that surgery is usually performed between ages 2 and 5, with one suture passing through testes and scrotum and attached to thigh; prevent pulling on thigh suture postoperatively; testes could reascend into the abdomen through the inguinal canal if suture disconnects

Points to Remember

Children have a greater percentage of body water than adults; because more of their body water is extracellular, it cannot be conserved well.

Children are more prone to fluid and electrolyte imbalance.

Urinary tract infections are caused by microbial invasion, chemical irritation, poor toileting hygiene, or incomplete emptying of the bladder.

Nephrosis and nephritis are caused by an autoimmune process against the glomeruli.

Glossary

Dehydration—a deficiency in body fluid from decreased intake, output greater than intake, or loss of fluids by vomiting, diarrhea, or diaphoresis

Enuresis—originally called bed-wetting; applies only to a child for whom control should have been attained; cannot be consciously controlled

Altered Musculoskeletal Functioning

Learning Objectives

After studying this section, the reader should be able to:

- Determine the nursing interventions necessary for children in casts, traction, and braces.

- Assess and plan care for a child with a musculoskeletal defect.

- Describe how musculoskeletal development from birth through adolescence predisposes children to various orthopedic conditions.

XI. Altered Musculoskeletal Functioning

A. Basic concepts

1. Bones and muscles grow and develop throughout childhood
2. Bone length occurs in the epiphyseal plates at the ends of bones; when the epiphyses close, growth stops
3. Bone healing occurs much faster than in adults, because children's bones are still growing
   a. The younger the child, the faster the bone heals
   b. Bone healing takes approximately 1 week for every year of life up to age 10
4. Orthopedic anomalies may interfere with the function of other organ systems

B. General assessment of musculoskeletal deviation

1. Assess function in the affected part
   a. Determine range of motion
   b. Note amount of weight child can bear
2. Assess quality of bone and tissue; is the correct amount of ossification present when evaluated by X-ray?
3. Determine whether all bones are correctly aligned
4. Determine whether musculoskeletal response is bilateral and equal
   a. Note if both arms and legs are used
   b. Note whether muscle response is brisk and strong
5. Assess child for pain; is he guarding a body part?
6. Determine the relationship of the child's body size and/or weight to the defect
7. Note whether the child has an adequate and even spread of adipose tissue
8. Note the child's autonomy and independence in terms of mobility and skills

C. Common orthopedic interventions

1. Cast care
   a. Be aware that chemical changes in the drying of a cast result in temperature extremes against the child's skin
   b. Be aware of discomfort to child as cast changes temperature
   c. Expose as much of the cast to air as possible, but cover exposed body parts
   d. Turn frequently to dry all sides of the cast; use palms to lift or turn wet cast to prevent indentations
   e. After it is dry, maintain a dry cast; wetting of cast will soften it and may cause skin irritation
   f. Smooth out rough edges of the cast, and petal cast
   g. Rub adjacent skin daily with alcohol to toughen it and prevent skin breakdown
   h. Assess circulation; note color, temperature, and edema of digits: note child's ability to wiggle extremities without tingling or numbness
   i. Assess drainage or foul odor from cast

      j. Prevent small objects or food from falling into cast

      k. Do not use powder on skin near cast; it becomes a medium for bacteria when it absorbs perspiration

      l. Before cast application or removal, demonstrate complete procedure on a doll, with the child's assistance, to decrease fear

2. Hip-spica cast: A body cast extending from midchest to legs; legs are abducted with a bar between them

    a. Never lift or turn child with crossbar

    b. Perform cast care as listed above but with additional measures

    c. Line the back of the cast with plastic or other waterproof material

    d. Keep cast level but on a slant, with the head of bed raised, so that urine and stool will drain downward away from the cast; a Bradford frame can be used for this purpose

    e. Use mattress firm enough to support cast; use pillows to support parts of cast, if needed

    f. Reposition child frequently to avoid pressure on skin and bony prominences; check for pressure as child grows

3. Traction: General information

    a. Traction decreases muscle spasms and realigns and positions bone ends

    b. Traction pulls on the distal end of bones

    c. The two main types of traction are skin and skeletal; skin traction pulls indirectly on the skeleton by pulling on the skin via adhesive, moleskin, and/or an elastic bandage; skeletal traction pulls directly on the skeleton via pins or tongs

    d. Keeping child in alignment can be difficult, because of his increased mobility and lack of understanding of the treatment

    e. Weights must hang free

    f. Nurse should check for skin irritation, infection at pin sites, and neurovascular response of extremity; prevent constipation by increasing fluids and fiber; prevent respiratory congestion by promoting pulmonary hygiene using blowing games; provide pain relief, if necessary; provide developmental stimulation

4. Bryant's traction

    a. The only skin traction designed specifically for lower extremities of children under age 2; child is his own countertraction

    b. Legs are kept straight and extend 90 degrees toward ceiling from the trunk; both legs are suspended even if only one is affected

    c. Buttocks are kept slightly off bed to ensure sufficient and continuous traction on the legs

    d. Traction is usually followed by application of a hip spica cast

5. Braces

    a. Metal hinged appliances that assist in mobility and posture

    b. Braces require good skin care, especially at bony prominences

    c. Braces must be checked to ensure accurate fit as child grows

    d. When applying full body braces to a spastic child, put feet in first

6. Milwaukee brace
   a. Extends from the iliac crest of pelvis to chin
   b. Used to halt progression of spinal curves of less than 40 degrees
   c. Must be fitted and worn over T-shirt to prevent skin irritation
   d. Can be used until child reaches skeletal maturity
   e. Must wear 23 hours a day; may be removed for bathing and swimming

D. Clubfoot (talipes)
1. Introduction
   a. Congenital disorder
   b. Foot and ankle are twisted and cannot be passively manipulated into correct position
2. Assessment
   a. Assess for talipes varus: inversion of ankles; soles of feet face each other
   b. Assess for talipes valgus: eversion of ankles; feet turn out
   c. Assess for talipes equinus: plantar flexion, as if pointing one's toes
   d. Assess for talipes calcaneus: dorsiflexion, as if walking on heels
3. Interventions
   a. Assist with application of a series of foot casts to stretch and realign the angle of foot gradually
   b. Perform passive range of motion exercises
   c. Assist with application of Denis Browne splint: high-top corrective shoes connected by a metal bar that adjusts angle of rotation of the ankle
   d. Ensure that shoes fit correctly
   e. Keep devices on as much as possible; stress importance to parents

E. Congenital hip dysplasia/dislocated hip
1. Introduction
   a. Abnormal development of head of femur and acetabulum; present at birth
   b. Occurs when head of femur is still cartilaginous and acetabulum is shallow; head of femur comes out of the hip socket
   c. May be from fetal position in utero, breech delivery, genetic predisposition, or laxity of the ligaments
   d. Occurs in varying degrees of dislocation; partial dislocation (subluxation) to complete dislocation
   e. Can affect one or both hips
2. Assessment
   a. Assess for restricted abduction
   b. Assess for Ortolani's click, which may be felt by fingers at hip area as femur head snaps out and back in the acetabulum; palpable during examination with baby's legs flexed and abducted
   c. Note shortened limb on the affected side (telescoping)
   d. Note asymmetrical skinfolds; the affected side will exhibit an increased number of folds on the posterior thigh when child is supine with knees bent; flattened buttocks appear when child is prone; these are from telescoping and dislocation

    e. Assess for Trendelenburg's sign, which appears when child stands on affected leg; opposite pelvis will dip to maintain erect posture

  3. Interventions

    a. Be aware that the goal of treatment is to enlarge and deepen the socket by pressure

    b. Gently stretch and maintain legs in an abducted position for at least 3 months, using triple-cloth diapering, casting, or a Frejka pillow splint

    c. Use Bryant's traction if the acetabulum does not deepen

    d. Be aware that older children may need hip-spica cast or corrective surgery

F. Legg-Calvé-Perthes disease (coxa plana)

  1. Introduction

    a. Ischemic asceptic necrosis of the head of the femur, resulting in degenerative changes from a disturbance of circulation to the femoral capital epiphysis

    b. Preschool and school-age children are affected

  2. Assessment

    a. Review history for a limp and hip pain or pain referred to knee, the first symptoms

    b. Assess for limited hip motion

    c. Be aware that it must be differentiated from synovitis

  3. Interventions

    a. Tell parents that treatment lasts 2 to 3 years

    b. Be aware that the younger the patient, the better the prognosis for recovery and the natural remodeling of the joint, giving patient an excellent prognosis

    c. Tell parents that child must avoid weight bearing until reossification occurs; this relieves pressure from femoral head and increases blood flow to area, thus preventing degeneration

    d. Be aware that bed rest with traction is followed by an abduction brace

G. Slipped capital femoral epiphysis

  1. Introduction

    a. Displacement of the proximal femoral epiphysis

    b. Displacement occurs during rapid growth period of adolescence; growth hormones weaken epiphyseal plate in hip joint

    c. Displacement occurs in teens who are actively growing or are overweight

  2. Assessment

    a. Review history for a limp

    b. Ask about pain in the groin or knee

    c. Note that foot turns outward during gait from limited internal rotation and abduction of hip

  3. Interventions

    a. Prepare for possible skeletal traction; may be followed by hip-spica cast

    b. Prepare for possible surgical stabilization and immobilization of hip with pin

    c. Teach patient and parents that weight loss will decrease stress on bones in obese children

    d. Maintain and teach parents about continuous assessment of opposite hip, since this condition may recur on opposite side

H. Scoliosis

1. Introduction
   a. Lateral curvature of the spine
   b. Commonly identified at puberty and throughout adolescence, especially among females
   c. Deformity ceases to progress when bone growth ceases
   d. Nonstructural/functional/postural scoliosis: nonprogressive C curve from some other deformity, such as poor posture, unequal leg length, or poor vision
   e. Structural/progressive scoliosis: progressive S curve with a primary and compensatory curvature resulting in spinal and rib changes

2. Assessment
   a. Assess for nonstructural scoliosis: when bending at waist to touch toes, curve in spinal column disappears
   b. Assess for structural scoliosis: when bending forward with knees straight and arms hanging down toward feet, spinal curve fails to straighten; asymmetry of hips, ribs, shoulders, and shoulder blades; X-rays assist in diagnosis; curve worsens with increased growth

3. Interventions for nonstructural scoliosis
   a. Shoe lifts
   b. Postural exercises
   c. Corrective lenses if problem is caused by poor vision

4. Interventions for structural scoliosis
   a. Teach child stretching exercises for spine
   b. Expect possible prolonged bracing with Milwaukee brace
   c. Provide emotional support to help child feel attractive while wearing brace
   d. Be aware that skin traction or halo femoral traction may be used
   e. Be aware that electrical stimulation may be used for mild to moderate curvatures
   f. Be aware that correction may involve spinal fusion with bone from iliac crest; instrumentation with Harrington, Luque, or Dwyer steel rods for curves greater than 40 degrees to realign spine

5. Interventions following spinal fusion and insertion of rods
   a. Turn only by logrolling
   b. Maintain correct body alignment
   c. Do not gatch bed; maintain bed in flat position
   d. Help patient adjust to increase in height and altered perception of physical self

I. Osteogenesis imperfecta
1. Introduction
   a. Hereditary disorder of connective tissue, involving bones, ligaments, and sclera
   b. Absence of normal adult collagen resulting in brittle bone, which is easily fractured
   c. Autosomal dominant disorder with different degrees of presentation
   d. Bone fragility that begins to cease with puberty
2. Assessment
   a. Note that bone age corresponds to chronologic age
   b. Review history for frequent fractures with abnormal healing; bones thickened, curved, or otherwise altered shape with repeated improper healing
   c. Assess for impaired growth and development
   d. Observe for blue-tinged sclera
   e. Check for bluish gray teeth from hypoplasia of dentin
   f. Assess for deafness from otosclerosis
   g. Be aware that spinal deformities often occur as the child reaches maturity
   h. Be aware that immobility for healing of one fracture may predispose the child to another
3. Interventions
   a. Provide gentle handling in all child care activities
   b. Be aware that pins may be used instead of casts
   c. Provide padded and soft environment

J. Juvenile rheumatoid arthritis (JRA)
1. Introduction
   a. Chronic inflammatory disease of the connective tissue characterized by chronic inflammation of the synovium and possible joint destruction
   b. Chronic autoimmune disease for which the genetic predisposition appears to be passed by HLA
   c. Disorder occurs in many different types
   d. Episodes of arthritis may recur with remissions and exacerbations
2. Assessment
   a. Assess for signs and symptoms of inflammation around joints
   b. Check for stiffness, pain, and guarding of affected joints
   c. Prepare for HLA studies
   d. Note that blood tests show elevated erythrocyte sedimentation rate, positive antinuclear antibody, presence of rheumatoid factor (IgM, anti-IgG)
   e. Assess with slit-lamp evaluation for iridocyclitis
3. Interventions
   a. Teach patient that stress, certain climates, and genetics can affect exacerbations
   b. Administer aspirin, corticosteroids, and nonsteroidal anti-inflammatory drugs

    c. Assist with exercise and range-of-motion activities

    d. Apply warm compresses, especially warm bath in morning

    e. Apply splints

    f. Stress the need for preventive eye care

    g. Provide assistance devices if necessary; encourage normal performance of daily activities

4. Monoarticular/pauciarticular JRA

    a. Asymmetrical involvement of less than four joints, usually affecting large joints such as knees, ankles, and elbows

    b. Monoarticular JRA may lead to iridocyclitis: scarring and adhesions of iris and ciliary body, resulting in cataracts and loss of vision

5. Polyarticular JRA

    a. Symmetrical involvement of more than five joints, especially hands and weight-bearing joints such as hips, knees, and feet

    b. Earache may result from involvement of temporomandibular joint; involvement of sternoclavicular joint may cause chest pain

6. Systemic disease with polyarthritis

    a. Disease involves lining of heart and lungs, blood cells, and abdominal organs

    b. Exacerbations may last months

    c. Fever, rash, and lymphadenopathy may occur

K. Duchenne's muscular dystrophy

1. Introduction

    a. One of many progressive muscular deterioration disorders that progresses throughout childhood

    b. Genetic; sex-linked recessive; occurs only in males

2. Assessment

    a. Assess for delayed motor development

    b. Note progression: begins with pelvic girdle weakness, indicated by a waddling gait and falling; then, muscle weakness and wasting progress to shoulder girdle; lordosis may occur

    c. Observe as child uses hands to push self up from the floor (Gower's sign)

    d. Note that child becomes wheelchair-bound, with decreased ability to perform self-care activities throughout adolescence

    e. Be aware that child eventually develops contractures and muscle hypertrophy

    f. Note that muscle biopsy shows fibrous degeneration and fatty deposits

    g. Death occurs from cardiac or pulmonary failure

3. Interventions

    a. Ensure that child remains as active and independent as his condition allows

    b. Perform range-of-motion exercises

    c. Apply braces, as necessary

    d. Provide emotional support and initiate genetic counseling

    e. Encourage continued activity and independence with self-care

Points to remember

Children's bones heal much faster than adults', because of the continued growth and development of the musculoskeletal system until after puberty.

Fetal positioning as well as heredity can predispose newborns to a variety of skeletal defects, such as osteogenesis imperfecta, clubfoot, and dislocated hip.

Rapid bone growth during puberty predisposes adolescents to numerous orthopedic conditions, such as scoliosis and slipped capital femoral epiphysis.

Juvenile rheumatoid arthritis is a chronic debilitating condition with periods of remission and exacerbation.

Glossary

Subluxation—partial dislocation of any joint

Talipes—clubfoot; the inability of the foot and/or ankle to attain correct alignment from twisting in any of multiple directions

Telescoping—apparent shortening of the affected limb, usually from dislocation of the femur

Altered Endocrine Functioning

Learning Objectives

After studying this section, the reader should be able to:

- Differentiate between Type I insulin-dependent diabetes mellitus (juvenile diabetes) and Type II non-insulin-dependent diabetes mellitus (maturity-onset diabetes).

- Assess and plan care for the child with Type I diabetes.

- Describe conditions resulting in hyposecretion and hypersecretion of the pituitary gland.

- Assess the alterations in growth and development from hyposecretion of thyroid hormones.

XII. Altered Endocrine Functioning

A. Basic concepts

1. Endocrine glands are ductless and secrete hormones directly into the circulation
2. The hormones are transported throughout the body and affect metabolic processes and functions
3. Hormone production and secretion is regulated through a feedback loop that interrelates many of the endocrine glands
4. Endocrine dysfunction may result from hyposecretion or hypersecretion of hormones
5. The pituitary gland releases growth hormone; the gonads produce hormones responsible for pubertal changes
6. The pituitary gland is called the master gland because it controls the release of other hormones; the anterior lobe affects growth, sexual development, and thyroid and adrenal function; the posterior lobe influences uterine contractions and produces antidiuretic hormone
7. Insulin production and antidiuretic hormone release are not under pituitary control

B. Type I diabetes mellitus (juvenile diabetes)

1. Introduction
   a. A chronic systemic disease most commonly diagnosed between ages 7 and 13
   b. Children with diabetes are insulin-dependent (Type I)
   c. A predisposition to diabetes may be genetically passed by HLA
   d. Insulin deficiency results from an autoimmune attack against the beta cells of the pancreas; this occurs approximately 1 week after an immune insult, such as an upper respiratory infection
   e. No insulin is produced and cells cannot utilize glucose; excess glucose in blood spills into the urine
   f. Increased blood glucose can act as an osmotic diuretic, resulting in dehydration, hypotension, and renal shutdown
   g. The body attempts to compensate for lost energy by breaking down fatty acids to form ketones with resulting metabolic acidosis
   h. Child appears thin and possibly malnourished
2. Assessment of hyperglycemia
   a. Be alert for rapid onset resulting from increased intake of sugar, decreased use of insulin, decreased exercise with no decrease in food intake, increased stressors, infection or cortisone use
   b. Ask about polyuria, polydipsia, and polyphagia; these are cardinal signs and symptoms
   c. Note weakness, fatigue, headache, nausea, vomiting, abdominal cramps
   d. Test for glycosuria and ketonuria using dipstick, Clinitest, Acetest, Ketodiastix, Tes-Tape
   e. Note hyperglycemia as measured by Dextrostick or blood glucose test
   f. Observe for dry, flushed skin

3. Interventions for hyperglycemia
   a. Administer regular insulin for fast action
   b. Give fluids without sugar to flush out acetone
   c. Follow treatment for acidosis
   d. Monitor blood glucose
4. Assessment of hypoglycemia/insulin shock
   a. From increased insulin use, excessive exercise, or failure to eat
   b. Assess for increased vital signs
   c. Observe for sweating
   d. Note tremors
   e. Ask about palpitations
   f. Observe for behavior changes
5. Interventions for hypoglycemia
   a. Give fast-acting carbohydrate, such as honey, orange juice, sugar cubes, followed later by a protein source
   b. Follow seizure precautions
6. Insulins
   a. Regular (clear/fast-acting): onset 30 minutes; peaks in 2 to 4 hours
   b. NPH (cloudy/intermediate-acting): onset 1 hour; peaks in 8 hours
   c. When giving both types, draw up clear insulin first
   d. Do not shake vial to prevent air bubbles
   e. Rotate injection sites to prevent lipodystrophy
   f. Make sure child eats at point when insulin peaks
   g. Increase insulin with illness, stress, growth, and increased food intake; decrease insulin with exercise
7. Complications common with Type I diabetes
   a. Life expectancy is shortened by one third
   b. Nephropathy is the primary cause of death
   c. Premature atherosclerosis with vascular insufficiency and renal failure are possible
   d. Retinopathy may lead to blindness
   e. Poor wound healing is characteristic
   f. Predisposition to infection is characteristic
8. Honeymoon period
   a. A one-time remission of the symptoms, which occurs shortly after insulin treatment is started
   b. Child can be insulin-free for up to 1 year (may need oral hypoglycemics), but symptoms of hyperglycemia will reappear and child will be insulin-dependent for life
   c. A last-ditch effort by pancreas to produce insulin

C. Deficient anterior pituitary hormone: Pituitary dwarfism
1. Introduction
   a. Hypopituitarism results in decreased growth hormone
   b. Can be idiopathic or from craniopharyngioma

2. Assessment
   a. Review history for normal birth length; then, assess for gradual decrease in height compared to peers
   b. Observe for short stature but normal body proportions
   c. Note that, physically, child appears younger than he is; usually well nourished
   d. Note bone age studies reveal growth retardation
   e. Note that mental age approximates chronologic age; normal intelligence
   f. Assess for delayed but normal pubertal development
   g. Assess teeth; dental anomalies at the time of eruption of permanent teeth due to growth retardation of the jaw
   h. Review family history to rule out genetic reason for lag in height
3. Interventions
   a. Administer growth hormone to help child catch up physically to his peers
   b. Treat according to mental age, not bone age or height
   c. Provide social and psychological support to deal with small size

D. Hypersecretion of anterior pituitary hormone: Gigantism/acromegaly
1. Introduction
   a. May be from hyperplasia of pituitary cells or a pituitary tumor
   b. May present different symptoms if hypersecretion occurs before or after closure of epiphyseal plates
   c. Disorder involves hypersecretion of growth hormone
2. Assessment
   a. Note that bone age studies are normal
   b. Assess for signs and symptoms of giantism if increased release of growth hormone occurs before closure of epiphyseal plates; elongation and enlargement of long bones and facial bones and accompanying body tissue; late closure of fontanels; proportional body growth
   c. Assess for signs and symptoms of acromegaly if increased release of growth hormone occurs after closure of epiphyseal plates; enlargement of hands, feet, nose, tongue, and jaw; thickening of skin and coarseness of facial features
3. Interventions
   a. Be aware that radiation may be used to retard growth
   b. Provide social and emotional support to deal with large size, especially for females

E. Hyposecretion of thyroid gland hormone: Cretinism
1. Introduction
   a. Thyroid regulates basal metabolic rate
   b. Decreased secretion of thyroid hormones results from decreased development of the thyroid gland or from medications that suppress hormone production; thyroid depends on dietary iodine and tyrosine to function normally

2. Assessment
   a. Evaluate for mental retardation that develops as disorder progresses
   b. Observe for short stature with persistence of infant proportions; legs are shorter in relation to trunk size, and neck is short and thick
   c. Assess for signs and symptoms of slow basal metabolic rate: easy weight gain; cool body and skin temperature; slow pulse; dry, scaly skin; and decreased perspiration
   d. Observe for enlarged tongue
   e. Assess for hypotonia
   f. Assess for delayed dentition
   g. Note blood tests show low serum T_3 and T_4 levels
3. Interventions
   a. Administer oral thyroid hormone (thyroxine)
   b. Administer supplemental vitamin D to prevent rickets resulting from rapid bone growth

Points to Remember

The pituitary and thyroid glands are vital to the physical and mental growth of the developing infant and child.

Type I (juvenile) diabetes mellitus is an autoimmune disorder that results in insulin dependency.

If the nurse finds a stuporous diabetic and cannot tell if he is suffering from hypoglycemia or hyperglycemia, she should treat for hypoglycemia.

Glossary

Acromegaly—elongation and enlargement of extremities and frontal head bones

Endocrine glands—glands that secrete hormones directly into the circulatory system for transport throughout the body

Honeymoon period—a one-time remission of symptoms of Type I diabetes, which begins shortly after insulin treatment has started and ends within 1 year

Altered Dermatologic Status

Learning Objectives

After studying this section, the reader should be able to:

- Assess and plan care for the child with a rash.

- Differentiate between contact dermatitis and infectious dermatitis.

XIII. Altered Dermatologic Status

A. The child with a rash

1. Introduction
   a. Children have thinner and more sensitive skin than adults
   b. Apparent birth marks in the newborn result from sensitivity of the infant's skin, incomplete migration of skin cells, or clogging of the pores
   c. Heat aggravates most skin rashes and increases pruritus; coolness decreases pruritus
   d. Macular rash: flat rash with color changes in circumscribed areas
   e. Papular rash: raised solid lesions with color changes in circumscribed areas
   f. Vesicular rash: small, raised circumscribed lesions filled with clear fluid

2. Assessment
   a. Describe the size, shape, type, location, warmth, and color of rash
   b. Note if erythema is blotchy or in discrete areas
   c. Assess distribution of rash
   d. Note if rash is dry or oozing; if hemorrhage or petechiae are present
   e. Note tenderness, pain, or pruritus; note any change in sensation
   f. Check the status of the hair and hair shafts
   g. Check history for allergies, contactants, new foods ingested, new clothes, wearing others' clothes, recent hikes in the woods
   h. Evaluate type of soaps used for laundry and body

3. Interventions
   a. Apply cool, soothing soaks of Burow's solution (aluminum acetate), or dab with calamine lotion
   b. Administer antipruritics; give antihistamines if rash is from allergy
   c. Distract child and give him projects that make him use his hands
   d. Keep affected area clean and dry; pat dry; use mild soap and water; expose to air
   e. Do not apply powder or cornstarch, as they encourage bacterial growth
   f. Do not use commercially prepared diaper wipes on broken skin; chemicals and alcohol in them may be irritating
   g. Prevent spread of infection by good handwashing; keep weeping lesions covered; teach child not to share combs or hats and not to scratch
   h. Prevent secondary infections by cutting nails and applying mittens and elbow restraints
   i. Suggest light, loose, nonirritating clothing

B. Contact dermatitis: Diaper rash

1. Introduction
   a. Rash in diaper area only; related to the moist, warm environment contained by a plastic lining
   b. Skin may be further irritated by acidic urine and stool or the formation of ammonia in the diaper
   c. Clothing dyes or soaps used to wash diapers may cause rash

      d. Additional contactants include body soaps, bubble baths, tight clothes, and wool or rough clothing

2. Assessment
   a. Look for characteristic bright red maculopapular rash in diaper area
   b. Note irritability since rash is painful, warm
3. Intervention
   a. Keep diaper area clean and dry; change diaper immediately after child voids or stools; wash area with mild soap and water
   b. Keep area open to the air without plastic bed linings, if possible
   c. Apply vitamin A and D skin cream (Desitin) to help skin heal

C. Contact dermatitis: Poison ivy

1. Introduction
   a. A contact dermatitis caused by the poisonous oil on the plant leaf
   b. A delayed hypersensitivity (T-cell) response; rash appears 1 to 2 days after contact
   c. Oils that remain on clothes and skin are contagious to others; the eruptions are *not* a source of infection and will not spread the disease
   d. Animals may carry the oils to humans
2. Assessment
   a. Assess for pruritus
   b. Observe for red, localized streaks that precede vesicles
3. Interventions
   a. Wash oils from skin with soap and water to prevent absorption through skin
   b. Do not touch other body parts until area has been cleansed
   c. Carefully wash resin out of clothes
   d. Apply calamine lotion

D. Impetigo

1. Introduction
   a. A superficial infection of the skin caused by group A beta-hemolytic streptococci; may also be due to staphylococci
   b. Highly contagious until all lesions are healed; spread by direct contact
   c. Commonly seen on the face and extremities, but may be spread on other parts of body by scratching
   d. Incubation period is 2 to 5 days after contact
   e. Common in children ages 2 to 5
2. Assessment
   a. Assess for a macular rash that progresses to a papular and vesicular rash, which oozes and forms a moist, honey-colored crust
   b. Assess for pruritus
3. Interventions
   a. Apply moist soaks of Burow's solution to soften lesions; remove crusts gently twice a day, and wash the area

b. Cover patient's hands, if necessary, to prevent secondary infection; cut his nails
c. Cover lesions to prevent spread
d. Administer penicillin for full 10-day course

E. Scalp ringworm (tinea capitis)
1. Introduction
   a. A fungal infection of the base of the hair shafts, causing hair to become brittle and to break off in the affected area
   b. Spreads in a circular pattern
   c. Is not contagious; complete healing may take 1 to 3 months to occur, even with treatment
2. Assessment
   a. Note spotty areas of alopecia
   b. Assess for circular area of scaly patches on scalp
   c. Identify by using Wood's light on the base of the affected hair shafts; reflects green instead of purple if hair is affected
3. Interventions
   a. Be aware that topical creams are not effective
   b. Administer oral griseofulvin

F. Pediculosis (head lice)
1. Introduction
   a. Common in school-age children who share clothing and combs and who have close physical contact, as in gym class
   b. Is not related to hygiene of the child or family
   c. Easily transmitted among children and their family members
2. Assessment
   a. Assess for lice eggs that look like white flecks attached firmly to the base of the hair shafts
   b. Ask about intense pruritus of the scalp
3. Interventions
   a. Use lindane (Kwell) shampoo, carefully following the manufacturer's directions, to avoid neurotoxicity; after hair washing, remove nits with a fine-tooth comb
   b. Wash bed linens, hats, combs, brushes, and anything else in contact with the hair; reinfestation occurs easily

G. Acne
1. Introduction
   a. Most common among adolescents from hormonal stimulation, an increase in sebaceous gland activity, plus the presence of bacteria that is normally on the skin, breaking down fatty acids
   b. The narrow channel between the gland and the surface becomes plugged with sebum, causing the follicles to expand into comedones, or pimples

     c. Acne is not caused by foods, poor hygiene, hairstyles, or emotions, although some of these factors can exacerbate the condition

     d. Acne is most common on the face, chest, and back

2. Assessment

     a. Assess for characteristic whiteheads: comedones that remain closed at the skin surface

     b. Assess for characteristic blackheads: comedones exposed to air (not dirt) that change color as they oxidize

3. Interventions

     a. Tell child to wash face daily with soap and water

     b. Apply topical vitamin A, tetracycline in older teens only, and erythromycin

     c. Promote self-esteem

     d. Address emotional concerns, and eliminate any factors known to exacerbate acne (this is very individualized)

Points to Remember

Coolness relieves pruritus, and heat intensifies it.

Scratching can lead to secondary infections.

Diaper rash and poison ivy are examples of contact dermatitis; impetigo, ringworm, and pediculosis are examples of skin irritations or infections caused by bacteria, fungi, or lice.

Glossary

Maculopapular rash—a combination of flat and raised circumscribed lesions with color changes, such as measles

Pruritus—itching

Vesicular rash—small, raised circumscribed lesions filled with clear fluid, such as varicella

The Child with Chronic Life-Threatening Disease

Learning Objectives

After studying this section, the reader should be able to:

- Describe coping strategies displayed by children with chronic illnesses/disabilities and their families; describe how the nurse can support them through this process.

- Assess and plan care for the major types of pediatric cancer.

- Understand staging protocols for the various solid tumors.

- Anticipate the psychosocial needs of children with cancer and their families.

- Assess the child's perception of death at various stages of development, and plan appropriate interventions when death is imminent.

XIV. The Child with Chronic Life-Threatening Disease

A. The child dealing with a chronic illness

1. Introduction
   a. The illness is relatively permanent
   b. It leaves a residual disability
   c. It is from a nonreversible pathologic alteration
   d. It requires special measures by the patient for rehabilitation
   e. It may require long-term supervision
   f. All disabilities/chronic illnesses can affect the physical, psychological, and/or social components of growth and development
   g. A chronically ill child who is in his normal state of wellness should be treated as well/healthy/normal and not sick/ill
   h. Assessment of the child's disabilities depends on the developmental expectations for each age-group and changes with age

2. Assessment findings of the chronically ill child and family
   a. Chronically ill infants are prone to deficits in stimulation
   b. Toddlers are deprived of autonomous behavior, becoming more dependent
   c. The children's fear of loss of body integrity is heightened by multiple testing
   d. School-age children often lose their sense of privacy and have their modesty abused; fear of death may be heightened
   e. Adolescents must deal with the label/stigma of the disability; may feel inferior and inadequate
   f. Children may rebel against treatments they have received for years
   g. The family's definitions of illness and expected sick role behaviors are important to child's response
   h. The family's view of their disabled child will affect the child's response
   i. Siblings may feel guilt, anger, fear, embarrassment; they may feel overprotective of their ill sibling or rejected by parents

3. Interventions with the child
   a. When child realizes he is different from his peers and understands that he has a disability/chronic illness, let him grieve at that time and at every stage of life when the disability interferes with developmental tasks
   b. Focus on child's strengths; provide him with as much autonomy as possible; focus on developmental age rather than chronologic age
   c. Mainstream or normalize child's environment
   d. Provide consistent limits, rules, and routines
   e. Provide therapeutic play
   f. Allow children over age 7 to participate in decisions about treatments

4. Interventions with the siblings and parents
   a. Allow the grieving process to occur; mourn the loss of the wished-for child
   b. Help family focus on the child's strengths
   c. Introduce family to support groups

B. Cancer
1. Introduction
   a. Alterations in cell function resulting from overproduction of immature and nonfunctional cells; tissue enlargement for no physiologic function
   b. Cancer can be life-threatening; can metastasize to distant locations
   c. Cancer can invade and destroy healthy tissues
   d. Goal is to achieve remission
   e. Pediatric cancers in order of frequency include leukemia, neurologic tumors, lymphomas, neuroblastomas, Wilms' tumor, and bone tumors
   f. A 5-year remission of cancer is considered a cure
   g. Any tumor is considered malignant until histologically identified, even if it is encapsulated
   h. Incidence of cancer increases with age
   i. Childhood cancers occur primarily in rapidly differentiating tissues, such as bone marrow
   j. Most pediatric cancers are sarcomas
   k. Childhood cancers grow faster because body tissues are normally in a state of rapid growth and high metabolic rate
   l. Cancer is second to accidents as the greatest cause of death in children
2. Assessment
   a. Be aware that signs and symptoms vary with type and location of cancer
   b. Assess for pain, abnormal skin lesions, fatigue, fever, weight loss
3. Interventions
   a. Assist with chemotherapy: a prescribed protocol including such drugs as cyclophosphamide (Cytoxan), methotrexate, vincristine, and prednisone
   b. Assist with radiation: one part of a multifaceted treatment program including surgery, irradiation, chemotherapy, and occasionally immunotherapy; used to prolong survival
   c. Prepare for possible surgery: performed for biopsy, tumor removal, determining extent of disease, and palliation

C. Leukemia
1. Introduction
   a. Abnormal, uncontrolled proliferation of WBCs
   b. Acute lymphocytic leukemia (ALL) is the most common type of leukemia and cancer in children
   c. Peak ages for ALL are ages 2 to 5; adolescents are more prone to acute myelogenous leukemia (AML)
   d. Highly associated with ionizing radiation, Down's syndrome, chemicals, and virus
   e. 90% to 95% of children with ALL achieve a first remission; 50% live 5 years
   f. 50% to 70% of adolescents with AML reach a first remission; 15% live 5 years
   g. Death usually follows overwhelming infection

    h. A child between ages 3 and 7 with ALL and an initial WBC count of less than 10,000 cu mm at time of diagnosis has best prognosis

2. Pathophysiology
   a. Blast cells are nonfunctional, cannot fight infection, and multiply continuously without respect to the body's needs
   b. Blast cells in the bone marrow may be as high as 95% and appear in the peripheral blood (normally, blast cells do not appear in peripheral blood and are less than 5% in the bone marrow, as measured by marrow aspiration in the posterior iliac crest [the sternum cannot be used in children])
   c. Increased proliferation of WBCs robs healthy cells of nutrition
   d. Bone marrow first undergoes hypertrophy, possibly resulting in pathologic fractures; then it undergoes atrophy, resulting in a decrease in all blood cells, which leads to anemia, bleeding disorders, and immunosuppression

3. Assessment
   a. Assess for bone pain from hypertrophy of marrow cavity
   b. Review history for infections
   c. Assess for signs and symptoms of anemia
   d. Observe for petechiae and ecchymosis
   e. Test urine, sputum, stool, and any emesis for blood
   f. Ask about nosebleeds, poor wound healing, oral lesions
   g. Palpate for lymphadenopathy
   h. Prepare for lumbar puncture, which indicates whether leukemic cells have crossed the blood-brain barrier

4. Interventions
   a. Prevent infection
   b. Inspect skin frequently
   c. Use interventions for anemia and thrombocytopenia
   d. Give increased fluids to flush chemotherapy through kidneys
   e. Provide high-protein, high-calorie, bland diet
   f. Provide pain relief
   g. Monitor CNS for involvement
   h. Gear nursing measures toward easing the side effects of radiation and chemotherapy
   i. Help child and family allay fears and guilt
   j. Offer hope, if appropriate
   k. Help child adjust to body-image changes
   l. Refer parents and adolescents with cancer to support groups

D. Hodgkin's lymphoma

1. Introduction
   a. A malignant neoplasm of the lymphoid tissue; patient has excellent prognosis
   b. Commonly seen in adolescents and young adults

      c. Usually originates in localized group of lymph nodes and proliferates via lymphocytes

2. Assessment
    a. Assess for painless, firm, persistently enlarged lymph nodes that appear insidiously; most common in lower cervical region
    b. Ask about night sweats
    c. Review history for recurrent fever
    d. Assess for weight loss without dieting

3. Interventions
    a. Assist with chemotherapy
    b. Assist with radiation
    c. Gear nursing measures toward easing the side effects of radiation and chemotherapy

4. Diagnosis/staging
    a. Definite diagnosis is made by computed tomography (CT) scan, ultrasound, or lymphangiogram in which dye is injected intravenously in feet (X-rays track dye as it travels up body and is absorbed by infected nodes)
    b. Stage I: involvement of single lymph node
    c. Stage II: involvement of two or more lymph nodes on same side of diaphragm
    d. Stage III: nodes appear on both sides of the diaphragm
    e. Stage IV: diffuse metastasis

E. Non-Hodgkin's lymphoma

1. Introduction
    a. Includes lymphosarcoma, reticulum cell sarcoma, and Burkitt's lymphoma
    b. Primary tumor arises in any lymphoid tissue
    c. Metastasizes faster than Hodgkin's and spreads beyond nodes into neighboring tissue

2. Assessment
    a. Assess for enlarged lymph nodes; most common in lower cervical region
    b. Note that symptoms depend on organ involved
    c. Assess for night sweats, fatigue, malaise, weight loss, fever

3. Interventions
    a. Be aware that the disorder has a poor prognosis
    b. Implement nursing care as for a child with leukemia (see "Leukemia")

F. Neuroblastoma

1. Introduction
    a. Tumors arise from embryonic cells in the neural crest that give rise to the adrenal medulla and the sympathetic ganglia
    b. Tumors usually arise from the adrenal gland but can also arise at multiple other sites; highly malignant
    c. If in the abdomen, resembles Wilms' tumor

2. Assessment
   a. Note location of tumor and stage
   b. Be aware that symptoms vary and are often from compression of tumor on adjacent structures
3. Interventions
   a. Be aware that treatment depends on location of tumor and stage
   b. Note that this cancer usually metastasizes before it is diagnosed; it has a poor prognosis, especially for children over age 2
4. Diagnosis/staging
   a. Definite diagnosis is made using ultrasound, CT scan, and a 24-hour urine collection to measure catecholamines preceded by vanillylmandelic acid (VMA) diet for 3 days (eliminate bananas, nuts, chocolate, vanilla)
   b. Stage I: tumor confined to the organ or structure of origin
   c. Stage II: continuity extends beyond primary site but not across midline
   d. Stage III: tumor extends beyond midline with bilateral regional lymph node involvement
   e. Stage IV: metastasis

G. Nephroblastoma (Wilms' tumor)
1. Introduction
   a. An embryonal cancer of the kidney originating during fetal life
   b. Average age at diagnosis is 2 to 4
   c. Favors left kidney; usually unilateral
   d. Remains encapsulated for a long time
   e. Prognosis is excellent if there is no metastasis
2. Assessment
   a. Assess for a nontender mass, usually midline near the liver; often identified by mother while bathing or dressing child
   b. Expect I.V. pyelography to assess kidney function
   c. Note any abdominal pain, hypertension, hematuria, anemia, or constipation
3. Interventions (preoperative)
   a. *Do not palpate abdomen;* it may disseminate cancer cells to other sites
   b. Prevent medical students and others from palpating mass
   c. Handle and bathe child carefully
   d. Loosen clothing near abdomen
   e. Prepare family for nephrectomy within 24 to 48 hours of diagnosis
4. Postoperative interventions include routine care of nephrectomy patient followed by chemotherapy and radiation
5. Diagnosis/staging
   a. Stage I: tumor limited to kidney
   b. Stage II: tumor extends beyond kidney but can be completely excised
   c. Stage III: tumor spreads but is confined to the abdomen and lymph nodes
   d. Stage IV: tumor metastasizes to lung, liver, bone, and brain

H. Osteogenic sarcoma

1. Introduction
   a. Most common bone cancer in children
   b. Peak age is late adolescence; rare in young children
   c. Usually involves the diaphyseal long bones; 50% of cases are in the femur
   d. Highly malignant; metastasizes quickly to lungs
   e. Survival rate is 60%
2. Assessment
   a. Sunburst effect on X-ray
   b. Pain and swelling at site
   c. History of trauma preceding the pain
   d. Bone marrow involvement may result in pathologic fractures
3. Interventions
   a. Reinforce that child did not cause tumor
   b. Anticipate amputation at the joint proximal to the tumor; some institutions remove only the bone and salvage the limb
   c. Provide psychological support, reinforcement of strengths, stump care, support through phantom limb pain, and preparation for a prosthesis after amputation
   d. Assist with chemotherapy

I. Ewing's tumor/sarcoma

1. Introduction
   a. Arises from cells within bone marrow rather than osseous tissue
   b. Occurs between ages 4 and 25
   c. Highly malignant to lungs and bone
2. Assessment
   a. Note pain and swelling at site
   b. Note that X-ray shows bone to appear moth-eaten
3. Interventions
   a. Assist with radiation and chemotherapy
   b. Note that amputation is not routine, since tumor spreads easily through the bone marrow

J. Graft-versus-host (GVH) reaction following tissue transplant

1. Introduction
   a. For a GVH reaction to occur, host must be immunologically incompetent; host must receive live, functioning, and immunologically competent cells; genetic difference must exist between donor and host
   b. The graft rejects the entire host
   c. Spleen, lymph nodes, thymus, and bone marrow are rich sources of immunocompetent cells that react against HLA of non-self antigens
   d. Occurs 10 days to several months after transplant, from cell-mediated cytotoxicity

2. Assessment
    a. Note increased bilirubin
    b. Assess for diarrhea
    c. Observe for rash leading to desquamation
3. Interventions
    a. Expect to suppress rejection with immunosuppressive drugs, such as steroids and azathioprine (Imuran)
    b. Observe for signs of infection; ensure protective isolation

K. The child's view of death
1. Parents' responses to potential death of their child
    a. Fear of the unexpected
    b. Anger
    c. Guilt at the thought that they caused the problem by not observing the symptoms earlier, not seeking health care earlier, or not providing a safe environment for their child
2. Child's perception of death is affected by language and cognitive development
    a. Nurse should give child facts and elicit feelings; allow hope
    b. Nurse should use language appropriate to cognitive age; do not substitute clichés, such as passed away, for the word death
    c. Child may seem unresponsive to the information at first; allow time for him to process the information
3. Toddlers
    a. Have no concept of time or space other than the here-and-now
    b. Fear of death only an extension of primary fear of separation from parents
    c. Can sense the feelings of those around them
4. Preschoolers
    a. Perceive death as only a temporary departure
    b. May relate death to sleep
    c. May fear separation from parents; may worry who will care for them after they die
    d. Possess a rudimentary concept of time
5. School-age children
    a. Understand past, present, and future; understand death's permanence
    b. Engage in games where they playact death; perceive death as immobility
    c. Possess a concrete understanding of causality; may construe illness as punishment for a misdeed
    d. Are afraid of pain and abandonment
    e. Are curious about the rituals of death; may ask directly about their death
6. Adolescents
    a. Express anger because they can't be independent or plan future goals
    b. May want to plan their own funeral
    c. May want to complete projects, make tapes to loved ones, or give belongings to others as a way of keeping part of themselves alive

7. When death is imminent
   a. Ensure that parent, relative, or health care person remains with child at all times to diminish fears of abandonment
   b. Discuss everyday life events or even death itself; encourage touch and hugging
   c. Encourage quiet, passive play that provided satisfaction in the past
   d. Help parents do all that they can do emotionally
   e. Include siblings and grandparents in the dying process

Points to Remember

Children with chronic disease/disability should be viewed as healthy, well, and normal when they are in their normal state of health.

The impact of a chronic illness/disability on a child continuously changes, depending on the child's stage of development; the child will need to readjust to the same disability many times during childhood.

Cancer in children occurs primarily in rapidly differentiating tissues, such as bone marrow and neurologic tissue.

Acute lymphocytic leukemia is the most common type of leukemia and the most common type of cancer in children.

Hodgkin's disease and Wilms' tumor in their early stages have excellent cure rates.

Nursing care for the cancer patient often focuses on minimizing side effects of chemotherapy, radiation, and surgical procedures.

The child's perception of death varies with age, depending on his concept of time and permanence and fear of separation from parents.

Glossary

Cancer—multiple and varying alterations in cell function resulting from overproduction of immature and nonfunctional cells or tissue enlargement for no physiologic reason

Chemotherapy—medical treatment with highly toxic doses of medications aimed at interfering with the mitotic division of cancerous cells

Chronic illness—one that is relatively permanent, is due to a nonreversible pathologic alteration that leaves a residual disability, and requires long-term supervision and special measures for rehabilitation

Remission—absence of all clinical and histologic signs of disease

Sarcoma—cancer involving muscles and connective tissues; more common in children than adults

Index

Notes